A Brief History of Love

What Attracts Us, How We Fall in Love and Why Biology Screws it All Up

Liat Yakir
PhD

WATKINS
1893

This edition first published in the UK and USA in 2024 by
Watkins, an imprint of Watkins Media Limited
Unit 11, Shepperton House
89-93 Shepperton Road
London
N1 3DF

enquiries@watkinspublishing.com

Design and typography copyright © Watkins Media Limited 2024

Text copyright © Liat Yakir 2024

1 2 3 4 5 6 7 8 9 10

Typeset by Lapiz

Printed and bound in the United Kingdom by TJ Books Ltd.

A CIP record for this book is available from the British Library

ISBN: 978-1-78678-823-8 (Hardback)
ISBN: 978-1-78678-825-2 (eBook)

www.watkinspublishing.com

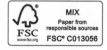

CONTENTS

INTRODUCTION

Philosophers have tried to define it for hundreds of years, painters have tried to paint it, poets have lamented over it, countless stories have been written about it, plays and movies have dealt with it, and yet love remains a mystery. So what can science in the 21st century tell us about love? Is it a thought? A feeling? An emotion? A need? Or an instinct?

Love must be one of the most complex and confusing feelings in the human experience. It is an integral part of our existence, and we remain preoccupied with it throughout our entire lives – from cradle to grave, from our prehistoric origins to these digital times. But don't take my word for it; do a little experiment yourself and type the word "love" into Google. About 13 billion search results will appear on screen, the highest number of results on the search engine. In comparison, type in the word "sex" and you'll get about 8.3 billion results, while the word "money" will give you about 9.5 billion hits and the word "God" has about 4.5 billion. These figures surprise a lot of people; during my lectures, when I ask which word has the most search results, everyone always choruses the same answer: "sex".

But the fact is that when people from different cultures around the world were asked in psychological experiments, "What is the meaning of life in your eyes? What gets you up in the morning?" 90 per cent mentioned the word love or a strong emotional connection that motivates them. However, not everyone is talking about the same kind of love. Most will say that it's love for their children that gives meaning to their lives (and children will usually say it's love for their parents until they reach the age of seven or so – after that, not so much), while others will describe a loving relationship as being what motivates them, and some will refer to bonds with family members and friends, or mention their love for a pet (especially dogs and cats) as being most meaningful to them.

It is strange that, relative to the level of our universal interest in love, the amount of knowledge we have about it is limited. The subject of love is not included in the school curriculum, nor is knowledge about it handed down as an oral tradition from parents to their children. On the whole, most of us tend not to talk about it.

When I asked the people closest to me, "What does love mean to you?" I received the following answers: my 13-year-old son, Milan, told me, "Love is when you want to hug and kiss hard." Eight-year-old Yoavi said that he "can't explain what love is in words". My friend Maya told me that, for her, "Love is a desire to be present, to breathe him, to contain him, something empowering. A desire to give, to assist, to be there for him." My sister-in-law Renana told me that, "Love is a strong feeling of affection, a desire to be near him, to see and fulfil his needs, even if a great sacrifice is required." Efrati, my best friend, put it another way: "Love is when the people I love the most have a crisis, illness or difficulty, I feel it as a physical pain in my body." My partner, Erez, told me that, "Love makes life more beautiful and instils endless optimism." And my friend Toval said that for him love is linked to two things: "A desire to be with the same person and a desire for him to be well."

It seems that the recurring motif in all these answers is that love is a strong and euphoric emotion, which arouses a desire for closeness and for giving to others. But what causes this feeling? Where is it created and which neurochemical mechanisms are responsible for it? And just what is an emotion, anyway? I want to invite you to join me on a fascinating journey into the depths of ourselves and to discover, once and for all, what emotions are, how they activate us, and the strongest emotion that motivates us at any age – love.

Exploring the Science of Love

I invite you to join me on a journey to explore the science of love. Together, we will try to understand what love is biologically, chemically and genetically, and which brain mechanisms produce love. I am a biologist through and through. My love for life sciences began in biology class at school. I had a teacher who knew how to fire up all the mirror neurons (more on which later) in his students and convey to them his love and admiration for the incredible complexity and beauty of nature. I completed my undergraduate studies in life sciences at Tel Aviv University, where I discovered the fascinating world of viruses. At the Weizmann Institute of Science in Rehovot, I continued my master's and doctorate studies in molecular genetics. My younger brother Asaf taught me the power of love. Asaf was cursed with a rare genetic disease that cut short his life – a disease caused by a change in 1 out of 3 billion letters in his DNA – and this has pushed me to delve into these lines of code which make up all of who we are.

While studying for my PhD, I went through a divorce after five years of marriage and two lovely children. It wasn't the first time. During my military service in Israel, I fell deeply in love with a tall, handsome man. He was my first love and with him I experienced my first kiss, my first sexual encounter and my first wedding. Immediately after leaving the army, I married him. But something happened after two years and I realized that we had been in too much of a hurry. We didn't have children together, so we haven't seen each other since. The second time round, things were more complicated. How do you break up a family? What do the children think about it – why don't Mum and Dad love each other anymore? I was suddenly surrounded by other couples getting divorced. We supported each other and created an alternative family network. During countless conversations, I noticed that almost all divorce stories are repetitive, as if everyone gets divorced for pretty much the same reasons and tells the same tale over and over again. After my divorce, I experienced several more-or-less good relationships and a toxic one, which contained warning signals I wilfully ignored, and was left with the scars as a result.

The personal journeys that I and my friends went through made me, as a scientist, want to try to understand what love really is. Biologically, because this is a language I'm fluent in, I get it that love is about hormones, neurons and genes. We fall in love over neurons. And a few minutes, hours, days or years after falling in love, our hormones kick in. But what happened millions of years before we knowingly started falling in love? Well, that's all down to our genes. Maybe we are actually captive to false conceptions about love and create an illusion that continues to be passed down from generation to generation?

The Structure of this Book

In this book, I'll begin by examining the biological basis of our emotions in chapter 1, before considering just what we are attracted to and why in chapter 2. In chapter 3, we'll be looking at same-sex love and how the biology of love applies to all human beings, regardless of sexual orientation. (With respect to this, the references throughout this book to differences between men and women refer first and foremost to the differences between male and female, and the dance between testosterone and oestrogen, regardless of the specific reproductive system a person has or their sexual orientation.) Next, chapter 4 dives headfirst into falling in love – particularly the role our hormones play. Chapter 5 asks what happens when two become three, and how having a family affects our love life. To answer whether we are programmed for fidelity, chapter 6 considers the impact of the sexual saturation effect, while chapter 7 explores the role of the alpha and males generally. Chapter 8 addresses the thorny question of whether humans are naturally monogamous. In chapter 9, I will be inviting you to speculate on the future of love, before chapter 10 sets out a prescription for maintaining a long-lasting relationship, if that's what we are looking for.

If this sounds a little detached and analytical, please don't get me wrong – I believe in love with all my heart. Without love, there is no point to life. I believe that to understand something means to be freed from it. Knowledge about the science of love will allow us to understand ourselves better and to create better, healthier and more loving relationships freed from the enslaving shackles of evolution. After all, most of us have never been taught about our operating system; we learn about it ourselves through trial and error. With this in mind, why not take the opportunity to save ourselves a lot of heartache, feelings of guilt, shame and unnecessary suffering?

We have reached a moment in human development where the old world no longer works, and we need to build a new one. Our previous models of love are not based on freedom and democracy. Evolution is not interested in the happiness of the individual but in the success of genes over thousands of generations. Nor were the empires and rulers of old interested in love, but in controlling people. We are now shedding that old world but have not yet put in place new structures, so we find ourselves in a time of confusion and helplessness. In order for us to know where we are going, it is very important to understand first who we are and where we came from . . .

CHAPTER I
THE HUMAN EMOTION MACHINE

The emoji that symbolizes love is a big, red, beating heart. We "give our hearts" when we fall in love and "break" them when love ends; but the emotion of love is not really created in the heart, of course – it comes from the mind.

The heart is greatly affected by emotional processes taking place in the brain, which is why we feel the heart beating strongly and heat spreading through our chest when we are emotionally aroused. We may also feel "butterflies" in the stomach when we are in love, because we have 500 million neurons in our intestines that are greatly influenced by everything that happens in the brain.

So, how exactly is an emotion created? To answer this, we first need to become acquainted with our brain, which has accompanied us since we were six-week-old foetuses and consists of about 1.5kg (over 3lbs) of neurons – or some 90 billion nerve cells – connected by trillions of connections called synapses. What passes through these connections forms who we are: our dreams, our aspirations, our memories and our emotions.

Our brain is not a single organ, but a collection of structures that have developed over 500 million years of evolution. The newest part of the brain, which is unique to us humans as the most advanced species, is the prefrontal cortex, which is located behind the forehead. In this area, 30 billion neurons (a third of the brain) accumulated some five million years ago, when we said goodbye to our cousins the chimpanzees. This is the area responsible for our higher cognitive abilities such as our rational thought processes, the regulation and control of our emotions, long-term planning, our conscience and sense of morality. This is also the part that matures slowly during our lives, and its development is complete only when we reach our late 20s or early 30s. However, we start to love and feel strong emotions long before the age of 30, and – unfortunately – there is no connection between love and rational thought. To discover the origins of love, along with all our other emotions, we will have to go back in time 200 million years and peel back the newer layers of the human brain to reach the older structures. There, between the temples and behind our eyes, sits the reptilian brain – the hallowed temple of our emotions – the limbic system. The ancient limbic brain contains several structures, which together form the human emotion and memory machine. This is the powerhouse that produces our entire range of emotions, including the basic emotions of fear, anger, sadness, disgust, surprise and joy.

The emotional brain is responsible for most of our behaviour. Researchers in the field of decision-making have found that 90 per cent of our decisions in life are based on emotions, resulting in so-called "irrational behaviour". It is important to note that the pathways in the "irrational" emotional brain operate seven times faster than the pathways in the rational brain, the prefrontal cortex. But how is it possible for 90 per cent of our behaviour and decisions to be irrational? Is this a complete failure of evolution, or is our definition of rationality flawed? To understand this, we must first find out what emotions are, what their role is, and what survival advantages they give us.

The Nature of Emotions

Emotion is a change in the brain's state of consciousness following the release of neurochemicals, chemicals that act on the brain. Nine families of neurochemicals are responsible for all of our emotions. There are chemicals for love, pleasure, anger, fear and so on. The very word "emotion" provides a clue: break it down into "e" and "motion", and it suggests something whose role is to motivate a creature into action – to cause a change in behaviour according to a need that arises.

Our fundamental human needs are to eat, survive and reproduce; therefore the strongest emotions that arise in us will be related to these needs. When we feel a negative emotion in response to certain stimuli, this indicates that a specific need of ours is not being met. The role of emotion in this instance is to make us change our behaviour and motivate us to act in order to satisfy that need and return to a state of equilibrium. Imagine you are sitting comfortably on the couch and an alarm sounds outside; your adrenal gland will immediately release a dose of cortisol and adrenaline (stress hormones) that will reach your brain, create a feeling of alertness and tension, and perhaps make you rush to seek shelter. The external stimulus (alarm) triggered the need (not to be hurt), which was translated into the appropriate chemicals, the stress hormones, which triggered the appropriate emotion (fear) in the brain, which in turn caused a change in behaviour (seeking shelter).

Our emotions are literally energy in motion. Energy that strives to be released and expressed in action. When we repress our emotions or don't express them, we imprison this energy, deplete our life force and become more exposed to anxiety, depression and even delusions.

Emotions burn themselves into our memories. As civil rights activist and author Maya Angelou once said, "People will forget what you said, they will forget what you did, but they will never forget how you made them feel." The chemicals linked to emotions increase the activity of the memory areas of the brain and the entire nervous system. Most of our memories are emotional, so we remember what was good for us and what hurt us when we encounter a similar situation again.

As our basic emotions are fear, anger, sadness, disgust, surprise and joy, this means there is one "positive" emotion (joy), one "neutral" (surprise) and four "negative" basic emotions. There is, moreover, a hierarchy of emotions: fear outweighs joy, jealousy outweighs tenderness, and so on, all of which suggests that the brain is programmed to focus more on what affects us detrimentally – on perceived dangers and unsatisfied needs – than on what affects us positively. An evolutionary logic lies behind this, since for most animals, the world is a dangerous place from the moment they are born. The chances of being eaten, starved, attacked or rejected are higher than the chances of resting on their laurels. Therefore, even if there is a risk of an animal acting incorrectly out of a gut reaction based on an emotion, such thinking makes complete sense in the long term (i.e., millions of years) in terms of the genes of the species, even if it's not always in the best interests of the individual in that moment. In general, genes are not particularly interested in the wellbeing of the individual but in the reproductive success of the species, and making decisions based on emotions is an excellent tool for their survival. It therefore follows that sexual love prevails over all other emotions in the hierarchy, including hunger, fatigue and the will to live.

Emotions as Communication

Emotions also form the basis of communication between us. We may register emotions first of all in someone's eyes – the window of the emotional brain. The chemicals of emotions affect the muscles of the eyes and face, and our brain takes about 15 milliseconds to detect a person's emotional state based on the look in their eyes. In contrast, it takes 300 milliseconds, 20 times longer, for the brain to decode words like "I love you". Ninety five per cent of the communication between humans occurs not through words but through feelings. Indeed, sometimes there may be a gap between what the eyes of the person in front of us show us and what their words say. For example, perhaps their eyes express rejection while their words convey affection. Our mind perceives the gap, which may confuse us: what do these signals really mean? It's perhaps not surprising that lovers' quarrels can sometimes resemble a conversation between two deaf people whose eyes and mouths are transmitting very mixed messages, resulting in complete confusion.

And, if that's not enough, emotions are contagious, as one person's emotional state can be reflected in the other person's brain through the mirror neuron system. The mirror neurons are a kind of mechanism that instantly connects us to another person, a fellow member of our species. This is the mechanism that allows us to participate in the feelings of somebody else, in addition to being able to understand that person on an intellectual level.

The discovery of mirror neurons by Professor Giacomo Rizzolatti, a neuroscientist from the University of Parma in Italy, is one of the most important findings in brain research in the last 30 years. Rizzolatti and his research team attached electrodes to the brains of macaque monkeys and recorded the activity of the neurons while the monkeys performed various tasks. One evening, a PhD student in the group, charged with recording the brain activity of a monkey eating nuts, stayed late in the lab and started to feel hungry. He went to the monkey's bowl, took a nut, peeled it and started eating. The monkey, mesmerized, looked at the person peeling and eating his nuts. When the student finished eating and glanced at the computer, he saw to his astonishment that 20 per cent of the monkey's neurons that were usually active while the monkey was eating a nut, were also active while the monkey watched the student eating a nut. This is the act of imitation.

Mirror neurons can be loosely defined as a group of neurons that are activated when we perform an action, and when we see others perform the same action. This also happens with emotions: for example, the same area that is activated when we experience pain is activated when we see somebody else experiencing pain, resulting in empathy, the ability to feel the emotions of the other. While yawning, smiling, laughing and crying in the company of others, we can see the mirror neurons in action. When we see a person stand in front of us and start yawning, smiling, laughing or crying, thanks to the mirror neurons, these expressions are recreated in our brain automatically, even before they appear on our face – and the face itself seems to react automatically, without control. Thanks to the mirror neuron system, the main communication between us is through emotions and body language – love gives rise to love, anger begets anger and joy brings joy . . .

Empathy tests show that women have higher empathic abilities and are more successful than men in identifying other people's emotions based on their eyes and facial expressions. These kind of differences in emotional communication between women and men, which we will expand on later, can make communication in relationships very challenging at times.

The Chemical Building Blocks of Love

The hormone oxytocin has been called many names: the love hormone, the kissing hormone, the hugging hormone, the cuddling hormone, the birth hormone, the breastfeeding hormone, the orgasm hormone and the social hormone – in all these situations oxytocin is secreted. Oxytocin is a short protein that is used as a neurochemical, a substance that transmits nerve messages both between the brain cells and between them and the body. It is produced in the emotional brain, in the hypothalamus, a small structure the size of an almond, which is responsible for regulating emotions, hunger, thirst, body temperature, heart function, stress and sexual behaviour. After oxytocin has been created in the hypothalamus, it is secreted into the bloodstream from the pituitary gland, which is responsible for regulating the amount of hormones after the hypothalamus produces them.

Oxytocin is secreted whenever we are in the company of people with whom we feel connected: when we look into each other's eyes, smile and laugh, hug and kiss, caress and make love; when we are complimented and when we are listened to (empathy); when we are told that everything will be all right and when we listen to music. Even when we fuss a pet, we and our furry companion secrete oxytocin in much the same way.

Amazingly, the production of oxytocin (and variants of it) has been passed down through 700 million years of evolution in a wide range of creatures – from worms to mammals. A high level of this hormone is secreted during birth, littering and spawning, and causes the uterus to contract. (In worms, the equivalent is called antimycin, an oxytocin-like peptide, which encourages egg-laying behaviour.) In mammals, oxytocin also plays an important role in breastfeeding: contact with the nipple stimulates the secretion of oxytocin, causing the mammary glands to contract. The high levels of oxytocin in childbirth and breastfeeding make the attachment between a mother and her offspring one of the strongest bonds in nature. Throughout evolution, oxytocin production has been perfected, reaching its peak in mammals, the most social class in the animal kingdom. When flocks, herds or groups of chimpanzees, zebras, buffalo, sheep or humans walk together from place to place, they secrete oxytocin.

Oxytocin is the common thread that links all our loves in life – for our spouses, children, family members, friends and, as we've seen, even for animals. This is why we use the same word – love – to describe a variety of feelings we can have toward others. The feelings that oxytocin produces are those of empathy, attachment, affection, trust, calmness, security and sexual arousal (depending on the context). Oxytocin also reduces feelings of stress and anxiety, because it activates the calming nervous system (via the vagus nerve), which triggers the body's "relax, digest and love" response, which in turn inhibits the sympathetic nervous system that activates the cortisol-dependent "fight, flee or freeze" response (through stress hormones). Every day of our lives, these two systems are locked in a constant struggle, and the friendship and love of the people around us are what helps us relax and deal with the pressures and stress we face. Evolutionarily speaking, our ancient ancestors relied on the stress response to hunt, fight and eliminate their enemies, and on the relaxation response of oxytocin to strengthen their social and romantic bonds, reproduce and build strong communities.

In order for us to remember those who do us good, make us feel safe and calm us down, oxytocin immediately triggers the release of dopamine – the hormone of pleasure, learning and motivation. When this pleasure hormone is linked to the love hormone, conditioning is created every time we are with the loved one, and sometimes we may develop a dependence on and addiction to our love for them or to love in general. Thus, we may find ourselves looking for someone to love in order to feel safe and calm, and life without love seems meaningless to us.

But besides giving rise to pleasant feelings of security and relaxation, we have already noted that the role of emotion in general is to change our behaviour and motivate us into action. Oxytocin basically makes us give up our selfish interests for the sake of another, and in the behavioural sense at least, this is the true meaning of love. When we love we put the needs of others before our own and share our resources. This is a behaviour that is not natural to us at all – we are all selfish creatures who are only supposed to take care of ourselves. Oxytocin makes us do the unbelievable: think about the needs of the other party, and sometimes even give priority to these over our own.

How exactly does this fit with the interests of our genes? Why should I give up what I have for the sake of others? What is the evolutionary logic of love?

We have touched upon how the highest dose of oxytocin in nature is produced at birth. The ultimate sacrifice is for the sake of our children, the offspring who will take our genes with them into the future. Similarly, it makes evolutionary sense to love and make sacrifices for family members such as our siblings and cousins according to their genetic closeness to us.

However, the most complicated and complex love of all is perhaps that of a long-term relationship. Here we see an admirable attempt by two strangers, without a pre-existing genetic kinship, to create a strong oxytocin-fuelled bond characterized by sacrifice and giving, in the hope that this will last a lifetime. In principle, the purpose of a long-term relationship and union between the sexes is primarily for the purposes of reproduction and raising offspring. The females and males of every species on the planet go out looking for each other every day, with the aim of maintaining a momentary or long-term attachment in order to pass on their genes to the next generation.

But what, then, is the connection between sex and love? How much oxytocin are males and females of different species programmed to produce in a relationship in order to pass down their genes to the next generation? When is there an advantage in casual sex with a random partner and when is a long-term relationship more desirable? Do genes prefer polygamy (multiple partners) or monogamy (one partner for life)? Under what conditions does monogamy develop, and are we humans by nature monogamous or polygamous creatures?

Despite all the songs, stories, plays and movies about love, we humans did not invent it. Love and the materials it is made of have existed on Earth for millions of years of evolution. Nor are we the only ones who make love and produce oxytocin not purely for reproductive purposes. Bonobo monkeys, like us, also make love for fun, relaxation and to strengthen the social bonds in a group. Nevertheless, why do we fall in love the way we do? It's time to take a closer look at the laws of attraction . . .

CHAPTER 2
THE LAWS OF ATTRACTION

I remember my first crush. I was in sixth grade when a classmate introduced me to the leading boy band at the time, New Kids on the Block. She had cassettes, teen magazine cuttings and life-size posters. We would lock ourselves in her room, listen to songs and fantasize about our tall, muscular, bronzed idols. I was in love with Danny Wood, who reminds me today of a combination of John Travolta and my father when he was young. But why are we attracted to some people and not others? What are the laws of attraction and how were they discovered?

In his twilight years, Darwin realized that despite the logic of his ideas about natural selection, specifically sexual selection, the way that females choose which males to mate with and which ones they find attractive is ultimately what determines the characteristics of all living creatures on Earth. Moreover, female choices can be somewhat arbitrary and not necessarily related to the traits that will increase the chances of a species' survival. Indeed, sometimes they can have the exact opposite effect.

For example, the penis is a very functional organ in that it greatly increases the chance that sperm will reach an egg and fertilization will occur. However, 97 per cent of male birds don't actually have a penis; they have lost theirs. So how did this happen? Well, the duck's penis, for example, achieves a stiff erection, ejaculating sperm at record speeds and over a considerable distance, which means that the male is able to fertilize the female forcibly even when she doesn't want him to. Female ducks, for their part, proved not to be particularly enthusiastic about either menacing penises or the males attached to them, and increasingly, they began to select more delicate males with smaller and smaller penises, until the organ itself became invisible.

Irrespective of whether he has a penis or not, the male bird of the blue sukhi species knows full well that if he doesn't work hard and present females with a fancy apartment exactly to their liking, he stands no chance. The bird labours to build a magnificent arbour of branches dyed blue from crushed blueberries. Then the female carefully examines the real estate, even though she has no intention of living in this blue-coloured residence. Impressed by his creativity, originality and innovation, she will accept the sperm of the male who has built the most impressive nest, and fly off afterwards to raise her chicks by herself while he arranges the nest for the next audition.

Originality is an important trait for females. Even in humans, the most intriguing male is the one who stands out from the crowd. An interesting example of this can be found in the spread of blue eyes in the human population. Originally, all humans had brown eyes, but a genetic mutation occurred 6,000 to 10,000 years ago in a gene that caused a reduction in the production of melanin in the iris, diluting the brown colour of eyes and turning them blue. But how did this trait spread from the same common ancestor? This is an example of sexual selection at its best. From a survival point of view, there is no advantage in having blue eyes, since one of the key roles of melanin is to absorb the harmful ultraviolet radiation waves from sunlight that cause mutations in DNA. According to the theory of natural selection, the mutation of blue eyes should have disappeared from the population as it doesn't contribute to the survival of the species. However, according to the laws of sexual selection, we have to assume that the blue-eyed ancestor who suddenly appeared on the scene enjoyed great success among the female sex precisely because he was different from all the brown-eyed people around. Most of us are attracted to those who seem special in some way – the one who isn't like everyone else. Our eyes love variety and novelty. We can witness the successful results of this dizzying form of attraction even today, thousands of years later, when 8 per cent of the world's population have blue eyes and Brad Pitt continues to win the title of the most beautiful man in the world year after year.

It's All in the Genes

Which evolutionary mechanisms are responsible, then, for the way we choose partners? A quick browse through Tinder and other dating apps offers an instructive glimpse into these complex mechanisms in humans, as shaped over millions of years of female and male evolution. Unsurprisingly, like other animals, we attach enormous importance to external appearances, signs of fertility and social status when choosing partners.

As previously mentioned, from a biological perspective, the purpose of an intimate relationship is first and foremost reproduction. Even if we are not of childbearing age and are not interested in children right now or indeed at all, our evolutionary coding is programmed to look for suitable partners with which to mix our genes and pass these on to the next generation, and our brain is therefore designed to look for good genes and to be attracted to them.

How do we identify good genes? For sighted people, 90 per cent of the information that enters our brain comes through our eyes. The optic nerve is the central information cable that transmits data from the outside world straight to the primitive emotional (limbic) brain, where the initial filtering is done by the amygdala, a paired structure located just behind the eyes and responsible for managing emotions. Within 30 seconds, the amygdala determines the initial impression of attraction – an instinctive and often unconscious emotional decision coming from the primitive brain, about whether a person "looks good", "doesn't look good", "passes" or "fails". The amygdala is mainly in charge of a process of elimination, ruling out negative options based on previous emotional memories and evolutionary codes. This small yet highly critical part of the brain focuses on the negative three times more than on the positive and its motto is "better safe than sorry"; this attitude means that sometimes we may end up being alone when we feel that we are faced by overwhelming choices, especially if we are steeped in past disappointments.

We receive most of our initial impressions about somebody from their face, which acts like a dating business card. Beauty in humans is not subjective but mathematical: the human eye likes to look at certain mathematical shapes and structures. Unconsciously, we look for symmetry between the sides of the face and the golden ratio in facial features. The golden ratio (or golden section) was identified approximately 2,500 years ago by the Ancient Greeks, who discovered that the shape of the rectangle is especially pleasing to the human eye when the ratio between its sides is 1 to 1.618 – i.e. the golden ratio. When this is found in the distances between the facial features, such as between the eyes, between the eyes and the mouth, the forehead and the lips, etc., our eye will find those features more beautiful. Men with symmetrical appearances do better on dating sites, and babies look longer at symmetrical faces.

Why do our brains translate a certain kind of mathematical facial symmetry into beauty and attractiveness? It is because this type of symmetry indicates that the embryonic development of the people we find beautiful was normal; every stage in their development happened exactly on time, without error, all of which indicates the presence of good-quality genes.

In cases involving genetic syndromes or problems in foetal development, there are sometimes differences to be found in the facial features of these individuals, which our brain translates as being less attractive. As mentioned, our brain's software is built to look for good genes for breeding purposes.

As a general principle, women are genetically attracted to more masculine-looking faces, while men are attracted to more feminine faces. Typically, female faces are characterized by roundness, smooth skin, a small chin, little facial hair, large, round eyes, arched eyebrows and full lips. This design is achieved by oestrogen, the female sex hormone secreted at its peak during puberty, which turns a girl into a woman. In contrast, a masculine face is characterized by broad jawbones, sunken eye sockets, a broad face, distinct cheekbones, rough skin and facial hair. This design is down to testosterone, the male sex hormone, which is secreted at its peak during puberty and turns a boy into a man.

High exposure to testosterone in the embryonic development of a man means that the ratio between the distance between his ears (the width of his face) and the distance between the line of the eyebrows and the line of the lips (length of the face) will be greater than those of women; that is, he will have a wider face. Women are generally attracted to men who have been exposed to more testosterone and exhibit larger width-to-height facial ratio (fWHR).

Similarly, exposure to oestrogen affects how attractive women appear to men. In a study carried out in England, researchers showed 29 people pictures of women taken at several times during the month, including during ovulation and menstruation. The participants did not know when each photo was taken, but they significantly rated the photos of the women during ovulation as more attractive than the photos of the same women during menstruation. Why was this so? During the month there are fluctuating the levels of oestrogen in a woman's blood. At ovulation the level is very high, and during menstruation there is a sharp decrease. Since oestrogen affects blood flow to the skin and water content in the body, the drop in oestrogen during menstruation causes the skin to look drier and thinner and the eyes less bright. This means that if you're a woman looking for a partner, it's a good idea to go on important dates around the time of ovulation and to go on fewer when you have your period. (Your hormones may mean that your attitude will be more positive then, too.)

In the same context, women wear make-up to give their faces an oestrogenic appearance of ovulation or orgasm, with bigger and brighter eyes, flushed cheeks, red lips, smooth and shiny skin – all signs of high oestrogen levels that stimulate the blood flow to the skin. The entire make-up and cosmetics industry tries to imitate the facial appearance and skin texture of women during ovulation.

What Do We Look for in Love?

Everyone is attracted to signs of health and fertility, but there are differences between the characteristics that are more important to straight women in their men, and the characteristics that are important to straight men in women. Various studies of these differences are currently being carried out on dating sites. These platforms represent a social experiment on an immense scale, during which a great deal of information can be gathered about the selection preferences and types of judgement used by women and men when it comes to meeting potential partners. For example, a group of sociologists at the University of Michigan randomly tracked 1.5 million interactions made by 1,855 people on a popular dating site. The researchers looked for the deal breakers for both sexes during their interactions on the site. They found age to be one: if somebody's age was not considered appropriate, there would be no interaction with that individual. Age played a more significant role for men in the survey, who consistently preferred younger women. For women the threshold criterion was height. If a man was 17cm (7in) taller than the woman, she would be ten times more likely to check his profile. On the other hand, a man would be three times more likely to engage with the profile of a woman 17cm (7in) shorter than himself.

Studies on various dating sites show that the issue of height is an essential consideration for women. Tall men are more successful in all areas of life: at school, in the military, at work and with the opposite sex. In humans, as in chimpanzees and other apes, men with normal testosterone levels are on average 15 per cent larger in body mass than women. Testosterone together with growth hormones during puberty lengthen the bones of a young boy's skeleton and build his muscle mass. So women tend to look for a man with a testosterone level that is on average about 15 times, but up to 100 times, their own testosterone levels. (Testosterone is produced in small amounts in a woman's ovaries and plays a role in the female libido.) In addition to a man's height, some women are attracted to large hands – they say it gives them a sense of security and protection. The size of hands and feet is also affected by exposure to testosterone and growth hormone during puberty.

A man's social status is similarly important in the eyes of women. In a study conducted in Singapore and the USA, researchers monitored the behaviour of approximately 600 male and female students, with an average

age of 22, in their chats on a dating site, and asked them to answer a questionnaire afterwards. The researchers found that the male students were more likely to reject women based on their appearance, whereas the female students were more likely to reject men based on their social status.

A man's social status can be expressed in a variety of ways, including ethnicity and country of origin, salary level, profession, degree, academic education, military background or achievements in sports. In 1986 and again in 1994, Professor David Buss from the University of Michigan examined the sexual preferences of 10,000 men and women from 37 different cultures from the West to the Far East – from Shanghai to Iran, from Germany to the Zulu nation in Africa. He concluded that men attach great importance to a woman's age and appearance, while women lend more weight to the parameters that indicate a man's social status, his ability to provide material resources and his level of ambition. The evolutionary explanation for this is, of course, that a man who is ranked highly in the social hierarchy will be able to provide sustenance and security for his offspring, even if he does not stick around and she ends up raising them on her own, which is the case with most species. Furthermore, if the man exhibits genes that suggest an ability to accumulate resources and power, then she wants those genes for her children, too. Whether we like it or not, behind many of our decisions, especially in the field of reproduction, lie the long-term interests of our genes.

Oxytocin, the Fuel of Attraction

Beyond the influence of the sex hormones, when searching for a prospective partner, we also look for signs of oxytocin, the love hormone. We can detect this through someone's eyes and facial expressions – their smile, laughter, kind gaze, empathy and sociability. As mentioned, the eyes truly are a window to the soul, or rather, to the emotional mind. Seventy per cent of our sensory receptors are located not in the skin but in the eyes, and within 15 milliseconds our brain can perceive the emotional state of another person through their eyes. The chemicals of all the emotions affect the six eye muscles; we can recognize joy, sadness, anger, fear, love, empathy, stress and many more emotions in the expressions of the eyes.

We can, of course, also perceive emotions through other facial expressions. The face has 43 muscles, which can create about 30 expressions. Oxytocin-induced facial expressions evoke closeness, trust and attraction. This is why people who are oxytocin "producers" – who smile and are funny, empathetic, full of joie de vivre and sociable – often have a mesmerizing appeal. It's a pleasure to be in their company, because they evoke a sense of security, relaxation and closeness by activating the oxytocin system in whoever is with them through the mirror neuron system. Oxytocin producers are also often considered sexually attractive, since oxytocin stimulates the genitals and increases sexual arousal.

In 1997, Arthur Aron, Professor of Psychology at the State University of New York at Stoney Brook, devised a famous 36-question questionnaire that can act as a handy shortcut for creating quick doses of oxytocin to break the ice on first dates. Professor Aron proved that strangers who used his questions on a blind date connected with and became closer to each other more quickly than those who alienated their dates with boring small talk. The questions in his questionnaire are intimate and deal with the essence of life; they raise emotionally charged memories, evoke empathy, touch on shared values and encourage honesty and vulnerability. In one version of the questionnaire, the participants pause every so often to give each other three compliments, one after the other, for positive reinforcement (in stark contrast to that other type of "blind date" – a job interview). Aron's subjects made connections and created trust because of the oxytocin produced during their honest, emotional, empathetic and mutually flattering conversation.

Body Shape and Attractiveness

After we have finished gathering information from the face and its expressions – happy or otherwise – in our quest to find the perfect partner, we will likely move on to examine their body carefully. Here, too, we will be looking for signs of fertility and health – signs of the sex hormones, oestrogen and testosterone.

Oestrogen shapes a woman's body by enlarging the breasts and buttocks, narrowing the waist, expanding the pelvis and hips, softening the skin, producing subcutaneous fat, and generally increasing the mass of fat in relation to muscle in the body. Testosterone, on the other hand, shapes the male body by producing muscles, broadening the shoulders and narrowing the pelvis to create a triangular physique. It increases the ratio of muscle to fat, roughens the skin and increases hairiness. Women and men, respectively, are attracted to masculine or feminine appearances that are the product of high exposure to testosterone during puberty in men and of high exposure to oestrogen during puberty in women.

The question is, why does this attract and stimulate us? What are the evolutionary advantages of the body structures shaped by the sex hormones in males and females?

Let's start with the structure of a woman's body. Our species has paid a heavy price for standing on two feet. The early reproductive success of the human race was not very impressive anyway compared to that of the animal kingdom, and declined even further once we started to stand upright. As a result of our transition to standing, the structure of the human pelvis changed. At about the same time, the human brain became larger, and thus an evolutionary preference was created for women with wide pelvises, which would allow the large brain of a foetus to develop in the womb. A body structure with a wide pelvis in relation to the waist is best for allowing a baby to pass through the birth canal with reasonable success. Let's remember that before advances in medicine, many women died during childbirth.

The reason why women's buttocks grow so much – as evidenced by the dizzying appeal of women with full buttocks, from Venus to Beyoncé and Kim Kardashian – is also related to a baby's brain. There is no other animal in nature that accumulates as much fat in the buttocks as humans do, because there is no other animal with such a large brain. In order for a baby's brain to develop in a woman's womb, she needs a lot of fatty acids to build that brain's nerve cells, especially omega-3 fatty acids, which are abundant in the buttocks. Under conditions of starvation, the fat cells in the buttocks do not react like other fat tissues; they are kept as an important reserve for the benefit of the baby during pregnancy and breastfeeding. This is why the fat from the buttocks comes off last during a diet. A female body structure full of curves and with a rounded butt conveys that she has the ability to conceive and give birth to healthy and intelligent babies – all of which stimulates the male mind.

But what is the advantage of the male body structure? If females in nature specialize in pregnancy and motherhood, males specialize in war. The fascist dictator Benito Mussolini put it this way: "War for men is like motherhood for women." In the natural world, many females of species instinctively look for warriors, meaning muscles and more muscles, and a large body adorned with horns or other war decorations. They want the biggest and most impressive alpha male, and if he is not available, then they will settle on those below him in a social hierarchy determined by physical fights between males.

Even among humans, men are still considered fighters. Armies of soldiers have determined, and still determine, the social order in many countries.

Throughout human history, warriors have received privileges according to their rank in the male hierarchy. Therefore, even in the 21st century, women are still attracted, consciously and unconsciously, to men with a body structure shaped by testosterone – the hormone of war and social status.

If Music Be the Food of Love . . .

What else contributes to sexual attraction? Interestingly, research on dating sites has shown that if a man is photographed holding a guitar, he will receive twice as many requests for dates, regardless of what he does for a living. In a French study, men who walked down the street carrying a guitar case also garnered more positive responses to their advances toward women than men who didn't carry one. But given that women are instinctively drawn to warriors, what is the connection between music and sexual attraction? Darwin was the first to claim that sexual selection is closely related to the development of music. The singing of males (birds or insects) conveys the same message to females as the magnificent feathered tail of the peacock, and that message is: "Pay attention to me, I am so healthy, talented and self-confident that I have no problem making loud, attention-grabbing noises and exposing myself to predators. I will not shrink from danger to woo you, my love!"

The late Professor Amotz Zahavi formulated this "look at me" message into the "principle of respect". According to Zahavi, the message should ideally come with a price that means the sender of the message can only afford to communicate it if he truly is as big, strong, healthy and successful as he claims. However, it is also interesting to note that since the reward for success in delivering the message is so important (i.e., the opportunity to mate) and the punishment for failure is unbearable, pressure has grown on males to cheat and cut corners. An example of this can be found in small tree crickets with weak voices who have learned to be deceptive. They look for a large leaf, gnaw a hole in the middle of it and half-crawl into it, thereby creating for themselves a kind of megaphone that increases their chirping artificially. The bigger male crickets don't need to cheat, because their chirp is loud and the females come to them anyway. Thus a kind of balance between males and females is created in nature, with the males perfecting their deceptive techniques during courtship and the females becoming increasingly suspicious and picky.

In addition to evoking the principle of respect, the sounds of a guitar stimulate the secretion of the love hormone, oxytocin, which, as mentioned, produces trust, connection and a sense of security. This is why music brings people together and has accompanied the social life of humans from time immemorial. Every culture has its music, which is passed down from generation to generation and forges oxytocin memories that connect us together and create a group identity. People who play and create music can have a hypnotic appeal, thanks to oxytocin. It's enjoyable to be in their company and (depending on the genre) the atmosphere may immediately become pleasant and relaxed, thanks to their music.

That said, a woman who is photographed with a guitar in her hands does not evoke the same reaction in men, although a woman who smiles in the photo and radiates warmth and joy will receive significantly more inquiries from men on dating sites. Once again, oxytocin is at work. As we know, it's nice to be in the company of oxytocin producers, who activate feelings of relaxation, ease and empathy through our neurons.

One of the selection strategies developed by women in turn is to value the opinion of other women about a man. In an experiment where a handsome young man walked down a street and asked passers-by if they wanted to sleep with him, 100 per cent of the women he approached shunned his advances. However, when a female "friend" stood next to the man and praised him, mentioning his caring nature and sensitivity, the rate of refusal dropped to 80 per cent. In the opposite experiment, where a young woman stood alone and asked male passers-by if they would agree to sleep with her, you can guess the results for yourself: 80 per cent said "yes" without waiting for a recommendation from other men.

So what, if anything, can we conclude from this? In order to be truly attractive, there is no point in worrying too much about your body (such as obsessing over your weight, size, appearance and signs of ageing). It is much better to invest in your own peace of mind and to approach life with joy, humour and an optimistic outlook, while tackling past traumas, getting rid of inhibiting behaviour patterns – and maybe also really learning to play the guitar.

At the same time, however, it pays to be aware of how senses over which you have little conscious control, such as smell, are very likely playing a role too . . .

Attraction Through Smell and Taste

A woman enters a closed room and sits down in front of a table on which seven closed boxes are placed. She opens box after box, smells what's inside and scribbles something on a blackboard. Right after she leaves, another woman enters the room and sniffs the boxes. This is not a focus group of a perfume company but the laboratory of Professor Klaus Woodkind, a zoologist at the University of Bern in Switzerland.

In 1995, Woodkind first performed the "sweaty shirt test", in which he asked 49 women to smell sweaty shirts worn by 44 men over three nights. The women were asked to rate the pleasantness of the smell and how attracted they were to it. When Woodkind examined his findings in depth, he discovered that the women were more attracted to the body odour of those men who were genetically distant from them with respect to six genes responsible for building the immune system. That is, the greater the differences between the woman and the man in these six genes, the more the woman was attracted to that man's body odour. The six genes in question are responsible, among other things, for building our personal proteins – proteins that act like the identity card of our cells, and which also create our unique body odour.

This phenomenon is not only unique to humans; female mice are also more attracted to the smell of males who have different immune system genes. Basically, this is a mechanism that uses the sense of smell to prevent incest. The evolutionary explanation for this is clear: the more Ma and Pa differ in their immune system genes, the more diverse their offspring will be; and the more diverse their genetics, the more resistant their children will be to disease. The difference in the genes of the immune system is actually an indication of the genetic difference between prospective partners. If a man's eyes are a window to his soul, then his armpit is a window to his genes, and genes, as we now know, always strive for diversity in the next generation in order to increase their chances of survival from generation to generation. It is clearly in the interest of our genes to encourage us to be sexually attracted to those who are different from us and not to those who are overly similar to us, such as relatives. Marriages between relatives increase the chances of passing on mutations and harming fertility in future generations.

The "chemistry" between spouses therefore begins with the chemistry of smells. The natural way we humans have developed to smell each other and test sexual attraction and arousal, without involving DNA tests, is through kissing.

"It's in his kiss," Cher sagely sang in the film *Mermaids*. Ninety per cent of the people in the world kiss, and even those who don't, like the Inuit, may rub noses. There is a whole science – called "philmatology" – that studies the kiss and its benefits. The purpose of the kiss is first and foremost to bring the noses together, to smell the partner's body odour and to exchange saliva rich in flavours and aromas. The kiss is actually an extremely important genetic health scan, involving the collection and analysis of multiple and valuable scent data, at the end of which a decision will be made about whether to continue sexual relations and the mixing of genes or not. Body odour gives us very important information about our genetics, as we saw in Woodkind's studies, as well as about our state of health and our hygiene. No fewer than 50 million bacteria pass from mouth to mouth during kissing. Kissing also reveals the level of our sex hormones – how masculine or feminine are we?

Our body odour is made up of a variety of chemicals produced by our cells, the bacteria that live on us and our sex pheromones. Pheromones are volatile chemical derivatives of the sex hormones, testosterone and oestrogen, which are released in sweat and secretions from the genitals. We cannot detect the smell of pheromones consciously, so when a test tube with pheromones produced in the laboratory is placed under our nose, it seems odourless; but the pheromones themselves reach the brain through the olfactory epithelium in the floor of the nose and bind to receptors that transmit information to the sexual arousal areas of our brain.

Professor Noam Sobel's research at the Weizmann Institute of Science showed that male pheromones extracted from men's sweat activated areas of women's brains, changed their mood and caused them to become sexually aroused. He also found that under the influence of male pheromones, women rated men as more attractive. Researchers from Sweden and Portugal found that female pheromones also induced a good mood in men, but this was influenced by whoever handed them the test tube to smell – on whether it was a man or a woman – meaning that the effect of the pheromones depended on the social context.

In the entire animal kingdom, from insects to mammals, pheromones are the main means of communication between species. At first, researchers believed that their effect on communication between the sexes in humans was not that significant, because we have lost the special sensory organ for pheromones – the Jacobson organ – that other animals have. However, we still have no fewer than 400 types of odour receptors on the olfactory epithelium in the nose. By way of comparison, we humans only have three types of light receptors in our eyes and two types of sound receptors in our ears. If with the help of only three light receptors we manage to produce such a spectacular visual world of colours, shapes and figures, we can only imagine what a whole world of stimuli is created in the brain by as many as 400 smell receptors.

There is much that is still unknown about the communication of smell between the sexes in humans, but without a doubt, we understand today that smell does indeed play a role in sexual attraction. Furthermore, there are those who have taken this knowledge out of the laboratory and applied it to real-life scenarios. After coming across an article about the "sweaty shirt test", in 2010 the American artist Judith Prays decided to set up "pheromone parties" to help single men and women find "the one", based on smell. Party guests were asked to sleep in white flannel shirts for three nights and to arrive at the party with the shirt packed in a sealed bag. The party organizers then wrote a number on each bag and placed it on one of two long tables near the dance floor – one for the women's shirts and the other for the men's.

During the party, guests were invited to go up to the tables and sniff the shirts. If you encountered a particularly attractive smell, you were to enter a side room, where a photographer would take a picture of you with the bag you'd selected. The image was then projected on a large screen next to the dance floor, and those who recognized their number on the screen were invited to look for the individual who'd fallen in love with the smell of his or her shirt. The next step was, of course, getting to know each other, kissing and completing the scent and gene scan.

The first pheromone party was held in Brooklyn and since then parties have been held elsewhere in the USA, England and other countries. While there have been no studies into how many of these pheromone party hook-ups have resulted in happy-ever-after couples, it can be assumed that the foundations for successful sex, based on pheromones, were indeed created there.

Opposites Attract . . . and So Do Similarities

Let's revisit one of the key roles that body odour plays: prohibiting incest. Social taboos prohibiting incest exist in all human societies. The Finnish sociologist and anthropologist Edvard Westermarck studied people's sense of repulsion about this topic and published a thesis describing it and other observations, *The History of Human Marriage*, in 1921. To explain the sexual rejection that brothers and sisters feel toward each other, he hypothesized that there is a "reverse imprint", which instils feelings of repulsion instead of attraction between brothers and sisters, and that this occurs at a very young age in children who live in the same house. This incest-prohibiting repulsion and rejection effect is named after him, the Westermarck effect.

Joseph Shepher's research on the residents of the kibbutz communities in Israel confirmed the Westermarck effect. A kibbutz is a commune based on socialist principles, where groups of unrelated children are raised in close proximity to one another. For many years, it was customary in a kibbutz for children to have their own sleeping arrangements, separate from the parental home. This shared accommodation meant that people in the same age group grew up together as if they were siblings, even when there was no genetic affinity between them. Throughout the course of human evolution, most of the people who grew up close to each other were probably close relatives; and even though they were not necessarily genetically related, the children in the kibbutz treated each other as if they were family members. The repulsion mechanism was activated and prevented members of the same age group from being sexually attracted to each other.

Shepher's research revealed a fascinating finding: there was not a single marriage between a man and a woman who grew up together in a kibbutz, where they would have shared bedrooms from infancy. The only couples that were formed were between people of different age groups, or between kibbutz children and children who came to the kibbutz later (usually after the age of four) and joined the group. The findings showed that kibbutz members who grew up together in shared accommodation treat each other like brother and sister. Also, the longer the cohabitation lasted, the greater the reluctance to hook up between the men and the women.

Further evidence of the Westermarck effect can be found in a study of a traditional type of Chinese arranged marriage known as shim-pua. In this type of marriage, unions were arranged between children from a very young age. Once both families agreed on marriage, the baby daughter sometimes moved in with her future husband in his parents' house. The two children basically grew up like siblings and a reluctance to have sex with each other developed. These marriages produced a much smaller number of offspring compared to other couples who met and married at a later age. They also had a much higher chance of ending in divorce and the percentage of mutual infidelities was higher than average.

Genetics, then, push us toward genetic diversity with the aim of improving the gene pool of the group. We are therefore programmed by a variety of means to be attracted to those who are genetically different from us. However, studies examining the success and satisfaction of couples over many years have found that those who are similar to each other in some respects manage to stay together for longer and are also happier than those who are very different from each other. The factors that determine sexual

21

attraction seem to be more complex than the obvious need for genetic diversity.

In royal families and in certain communities in Kazakhstan and Ethiopia, it was and still is the practice to make sure that there is no blood relation between the groom and the bride going back seven generations. This practice was established at around the same time in different parts of the world and it seems that behind it lies a calculation of some sort relating to the required degree of genetic diversity. The ideal situation, in terms of providing healthy genes for the next generation, is that there should be some variation between the genes of partners – but not too much variation. While it's best to avoid sexual congress between genetic relatives, which increases the likelihood of passing on mutations that will reduce fertility in the long term, it is also preferable to avoid there being too great a genetic difference, meaning that the genes of both partners will still belong to the same broad genetic group – the same people, the same race, and so on. Mathematically, that works out at about seven generations.

Most human societies exhibit a strong preoccupation – through their customs, prohibitions and laws – with the reproduction of the members of that culture and especially with regulating the reproductive choices of women, which may often be controlled by the men in their family. But even without customs rooted in culture and draconian social prohibitions, it turns out that our brain performs much the same genetic kinship calculations by itself when we meet a potential partner. Proximity calculations are carried out by each of us unconsciously, involving old and new algorithms, and at the end a decision is reached about whether or not everything "clicks" with a potential partner.

First, in order to identify the degree of genetic closeness, we examine the differences between us and a potential partner in terms of our skin colour, facial structure, eyes, mother tongue, accent, favourite foods and clothing style. All these parameters point to our own ethnic affiliation and to the pool of genes that the potential partner belongs to. The human face consists of a complex pattern of features and is our primary means of distinguishing people. Studies have shown that people are better at remembering the faces of people with the same ethnic origins as their own. As mentioned, we attach enormous importance to the face in terms of its attractiveness. The structure of the face has a strong genetic basis and is a kind of advertisement about the origins of our genes and our genetic qualities. Facial resemblance between spouses is a phenomenon that has been observed in various different cultures. In a 2013 study, people were shown photos of their partner that had been altered to contain either some of the participant's own facial features or a stranger's face. Time after time, the participants chose the facial composition that contained their own characteristics as being more attractive than the facial composition that contained foreign facial characteristics.

This mechanism of similar preference is called "similar selection", and it is not unique to us humans but exists throughout the animal kingdom. For example, a female light blue thrush chooses to mate with a light blue male, while a dark blue female thrush stays longer with a dark blue male. A large Japanese toad often chooses to mate with a male Japanese toad of a similar size to her own. In addition to this, there are various species of lizard in which the females clearly choose the males that look outwardly similar to them, and when researchers tested the genetic kinship by sequencing their genomes (a genome is the sum total of our hereditary genetic material), they did find a distinct similarity between them.

Genetic studies have also been conducted in humans in which the genetic and physical traits of married couples were compared, and genetic similarity was found between spouses. The researchers claim that our personal and socio-cultural tendency to choose partners who resemble us significantly influenced the evolution of the human genome. The study was conducted in 2017 in Australia, when geneticists analysed a database of 24,000 married couples, including information about their physical and genetic traits. The researchers compared genetic markers of characteristics such as height and weight/height ratio (body mass index or BMI) and found a strong statistical correlation between the genetic markers of the married couples.

How does the mechanism of "similarity preference" work at a brain level? While the prefrontal cortex calculates the genetic proximity of a potential partner to us through their facial structure, skin colour and other characteristics, the emotional brain analyses what feelings this evokes in us, and how familiar we feel he or she is. Sometimes we may sense a kind of chemistry with a certain person that will instil in us feelings of trust and ease, of feeling at home with them, as if we already know each other, and this sense of ease will not arise with another person. This chemistry is actually related to the love hormone oxytocin and the memories imprinted in our minds by this hormone, which come up again and again when we choose partners.

Imprinting and the Foundations of Attraction

Visual images of the people who took care of us during the first five years of our lives are fixed in our minds through the action of oxytocin on the memory areas of the brain, in a process called imprinting. Imprinting entails forming a strong attachment to the images of the first people we saw when we were born, who took care of us and (hopefully) showered us with love at the start of life. Usually, these are first and foremost the images of our parents when they were younger, but perhaps also brothers and sisters, uncles, aunts and grandparents. After puberty, when we meet potential partners, the memories come alive of all those caring figures of the opposite sex who showered us with love during childhood. This does not mean that we will immediately fall in love with anyone who resembles our father or mother, but it is possible that certain qualities – external or internal – of a potential partner will bring to life oxytocin memories associated with the people who loved us in our childhood and make us feel a sense of closeness and security in their company more than in the company of others.

The imprinting process takes place in the brains of almost all animals – reptiles, birds and mammals – immediately after they emerge into the world. The Austrian researcher Konrad Lorenz was the first to define the phenomenon in the 1930s. He noticed that goose chicks he raised in his house followed him everywhere because he was the first moving creature they saw. Lorenz also realized that in order for them to get into the water and swim, he had to get in there first. The chicks were imprinted by Lorenz and there was no way to change that. From then on, they preferred him and ignored their own kind.

The imprinting wiring is so rigid and powerful that it can also affect a couple's attraction to each other, as was shown in a roundabout way by an experiment carried out in 1999 by researchers at the University of Oxford. The researchers took a newborn baby goat, separated it immediately from its biological mother and transferred it to an adoptive mother, a ewe who had just given birth, to raise it as if it were her own. When the young goat reached sexual maturity and became a full-fledged adult, the researchers asked themselves who he would chase and court. Would he run after female goats or female sheep? The goat only chased after sheep and ignored the female goats. The experiment showed that the imprint of the "mother sheep" wired into the young goat's brain overrode the evolutionary wiring for sexual attraction to the pheromones of the female goat. (Remember that pheromones are odorants unique to a species, found in high concentrations in secretions from the genitals, especially during oestrus.) Researchers repeated these adoption experiments with newly hatched chicks raised by mother ducks, as well as with other animals, and the results were consistent.

The imprinting and attachment formed at the beginning of life to a mother figure outweighs the attraction to sexual pheromones later in life.

In order to examine the effect of imprinting on the choice of their partners by humans, in 2002 researchers from Hungary asked nine impartial individuals to look for similarities between a wide range of pictures of young and old women. The participants didn't receive any information about the women in the photographs, yet at a significantly higher than random rate, they made connections between pictures of women who were brides and those of their mothers-in-law. This suggests that the men who were married to these women were more attracted to girls who somehow reminded them of their mothers and that they then wed them. This was also found to be true of women's attraction to partners who remind them of their fathers. The participants in the study paired pictures of fathers with pictures of the husbands chosen by their daughters, without having any prior knowledge of the connections between the older and younger men. Moreover, the attraction to characteristics in a partner that remind us of our parent of the opposite sex is not just visually informed; there are studies that show the similarity of a spouse to a parent with respect to their personal traits is often more significant than their outer appearance.

We understand today that the laws of attraction are complex and confusing. We are sexually attracted to the different, but end up staying more often with the same. Eighty-six per cent of those looking for love state that they are looking for someone with opposite traits to their own, but research shows that the more similar partners are in their physical and genetic traits, the more likely they will stay together. Science tells us that the "ignition", "chemistry" and "click" processes occur in the unconscious areas of the brain and are influenced by a variety of genetic, evolutionary, familial, psychological, social and cultural factors. Many different types of hardwiring are involved in these processes, some of which were formed by evolution and some of which were shaped by the people who loved us from the moment we entered the world, when they burned themselves into our memories. Our different types of hardwiring can be contradictory and confusing, to the point where they may prevent us from settling on one person and creating a stable relationship. For example, a person may stir up feelings of closeness and familiarity in us but not sexual attraction, whereas at other times the sexual attraction is strong but a sense of ease and stability isn't there. Occasionally the mind plays tricks on us and we can find ourselves caught up in a constant search for the one person with whom we will feel that everything is perfect, the one who will activate all our sexual, family, social and genetic hardwiring and match all its parameters. But what is the real chance of finding "the one"?

Do Birth Control Pills Effect Sexual Attraction?

Certainly, the chances of discovering your soulmate may be limited if your body thinks it's already done the job for you.

The contraceptive pill that entered our lives in 1960 was considered to be revolutionary and one of the most important inventions ever in the history of women. The pill gave women sexual freedom, control over their bodies and more gender equality. It prevented unwanted pregnancies and the abortions and complications associated with them.

The pill prevents ovulation (the release of the egg from the ovary) by suppressing the secretion of certain hormones from the brain, which act on the ovaries. It contains oestrogen alongside progestin (a synthetic derivative of the hormone progesterone), which reduce the secretion of ovulation hormones and thus suppress the development of follicles in the ovary. As a result, ovulation – the process during which a ripe egg hatches from one of the follicles, migrates toward the uterus and becomes available for fertilization – is prevented. The pill actually cancels a woman's menstrual cycle and ovulation.

One hundred women aged between 18 and 35 participated in a study by Craig Roberts at Newcastle University in England. The women had to rate their preference for six body odour samples taken from different men. At the beginning of the experiment, none of the women took birth control pills, but after three months the women were again given the same choice between six odour samples, only this time 40 of the women had been taking the contraceptive pill for two months.

With respect to the women who didn't take the pill at all, the results didn't show a clear preference for the smells of men with similar or different MHC molecules. But for those women who started taking the pill, this changed. These women suddenly preferred the smells of men whose MHC molecules were more similar to their own. That is, the women's preference under the influence of the pill changed to men who were more genetically similar to them. In a study in Switzerland in the 1990s, Klaus Wadkins discovered similar findings in women who took the pill.

The explanation for this is that the pill puts a woman's body into a hormonal state of pregnancy (during which she will not ovulate), and during pregnancy, there is no reason for her to search for a partner for the purposes of reproduction. Nor is there any pressure from an evolutionary point of view for a pregnant woman to select a partner, and if there is some form of pressure, then it is toward connecting with people who are genetically closer to her, because they will be more helpful in taking care of the offspring. The pill therefore has the unintended effect of simulating pregnancy and all that this entails at precisely the moment when a woman is potentially looking for a partner.

Another effect of the pill due to the suppression of ovulation hormones is on women's sex drive. The hormones found in oestrogen and progestin contraceptive pills inhibit the production of testosterone, which directly affects the sex drive and amount of pleasure that women feel during intercourse. In 2006, a study in Boston involving 124 women examined the relationship between the female libido and the pill, and found that women who used the pill reported a lower level of libido than women who did not use it and that the level of testosterone in their bodies decreased.

In 2007, evolutionary psychologist Geoffrey Miller from the University of New Mexico, along with Brent Jordan and Joshua Tybur, conducted a study to examine the effect of ovulation on strippers' incomes. They collected the information through a website set up for this purpose and found that during ovulation the strippers earned an average of $30 an hour more than menstruating women, and $15 more than women who were not menstruating or ovulating. The women who took birth control pills earned significantly less than those women with a natural cycle.

Although we women, unlike other female mammals, hide our oestrous period, i.e., ovulation, the hormones that are secreted during this time still affect our appearance, smell and sexual appeal in significant ways. It seems that contraceptive pills inhibit the body's natural secretion of hormones with many consequences that still need to be investigated more deeply.

Even the use of medication to combat anxiety impacts the love life and sexuality of women and men, due to the effects of these on the secretion of hormones. SSRIs (serotonin selective reabsorption inhibitors) were first used in the early 1990s to treat depression and anxiety. Since then the psychiatric pill industry has developed into a global market, with revenues of more than 40 billion dollars a year. These drugs inhibit the process of reabsorption of serotonin, the happy hormone, in the brain, so that serotonin remains longer in the synapses. However, one of the known side effects is the reduction in sex drive, which affects up to 70 per cent of users.

Serotonin is partly responsible for our mood. It contributes to uplifting, positive feelings and lowers levels of the stress hormone cortisol. But the same drugs also harm the desire for sex and sexual function and the ability to orgasm. While the damage that these drugs do to sexual function is well known, it now transpires that while an individual's mood rises, their feelings of love fade. According to the findings of the anthropologist Dr Helen Fisher, the drugs that act on serotonin levels interfere with brain activity involved in love and emotional connection. When the sexual urge is damaged, the ability to love is also damaged.

As mentioned, the ability to create an emotional connection, to love, comprises three stages, with different hormones playing a role in each stage. Initial attraction is activated by the sex hormones; falling in love is driven by dopamine, adrenaline and serotonin; and, finally, attachment is mediated by the love hormone oxytocin. Raising serotonin levels through antidepressants may not only harm sexual desire and function, but also adversely affect the three stages that lead to long-term love.

The Mathematics of Love

Perhaps the Disney movies and the fairy tales that we grew up with are responsible for creating the illusion that each and every one of us has a soulmate waiting for us somewhere, our very own Prince Charming or Sleeping Beauty. The one who fits all our parameters and with whom we will live happily ever after. Beliefs about twin souls are also common in Asian cultures. According to Chinese mythology (and a common thread in Japanese and Korean myth, too), when a baby is born, a long red thread is tied to its little finger connecting it with its twin soul. During its life, the thread gets tangled and tied and the two souls may never meet, but the bond between them will never break and cannot be broken. This is the bond of destiny between soulmates. The person responsible for connecting the red threads in Chinese mythology is the god of matches, Yue Lao. Similarly, in Judaism, there is a belief that each person's marriage is determined by a decree from heaven that cannot be changed.

Myths aside, most of us roam the world looking for some kind of perfect figure who we believe is the perfect match meant for us, and eventually will come into our lives. We often have a mental shopping list of our intended: they should be clever, educated, sexy and good-looking, funny, spontaneous, established and successful, ambitious, sensual lovers, kind-hearted, and also be good parents. In fact, that's at least seven different people, not one. And women's shopping lists are even longer than men's lists. Women on the dating site OK Cupid rated 80 per cent of the men's profiles as "below average". Is it any wonder that so many women all over the world feel frustrated and full of despair when it comes to finding love?

If love is destiny, then what are the real chances of our finding a soulmate? Is it possible to quantify fate? For this purpose we will once again enlist the help of mathematics, the mother of sciences. Rachel Riley, mathematician and British TV star, teamed up with mathematicians from the University of Bath to calculate the probability of someone finding a perfect match in England based on 18 parameters. To that end, they used the Drake equation, which was developed by the astronomer Frank Drake in the 1960s, and with the help of which he calculated the probability of finding intelligent life in the universe. The equation is a product of a series of fractions that represent several variables related to the development of life on planets.

Riley and her team replaced the variables in the Drake equation with variables relating to finding a suitable partner in England. They included the following variables in the equation:

- the part of the population who are of the appropriate gender (39 per cent)
- those who were the right age (17 per cent), as people generally prefer partners whose age falls within an average range of six years of their own
- those who have a suitable married status (e.g., single/divorced/widowed)
- those who have a suitable education
- those who have similar worldviews
- those who are suitable in terms of personality traits (40 per cent)
- those who have similar interests
- the chance that the attraction will be mutual (18 per cent)
- additional factors

The result of the calculation for England was 84,440. That is, out of the population of England, which numbers approximately 47 million people, there are 84,440 people out there who will fit you in all these parameters. This means that your chances of finding "the one" are 1 in 562 or 0.17 per cent! Ten times better than the odds of becoming a millionaire in England, which is 1 in 55, and about as likely as humanity becoming extinct next year. Your age is also a factor in your chances of finding the right partner. Before the age of 24, the odds are as low as 1 in 1,024, while senior citizens stand the best chance at 1 in 304.

What the maths teaches us is that we should ignore Disney movies and stop looking for "the one". Life is just a game of probabilities, and the more we add variables and tighten our criteria, the smaller the probability of finding our "perfect" relationship becomes. When it comes to finding long-term love, flexibility is a must. The number of parameters on the shopping list should be reduced, our requirements should be more realistic and the most important features prioritized.

So what are the lines that cannot be crossed? In what ways can the probability of finding a suitable partner be increased? According to researchers, here are some activities that increase the chances of finding "the one":

- Getting to know people through friends and colleagues increases them by 16 per cent.
- Joining a gym increases them by 15 per cent.
- Getting to know each other through shared hobbies increases them by 11 per cent.
- Sitting in a bar by 9 per cent.
- Meeting friends of friends increases them by 8 per cent (but getting to know people through family members only by 1 per cent).
- Registering on dating sites increases the chances by 17 per cent, due to the massive expansion of your pool of possibilities.

From a mathematical point of view, it is easier to find a suitable partner in the digital age, since the dating sites have significantly increased our options. On the other hand, our brains were shaped in the prehistoric era, and we are not capable of analysing so much data about so many people all at the same time.

It's interesting to note that in the equation formulated by Riley and her colleagues, one of the variables that significantly decreases the chance of finding a suitable partner is that of mutual attraction. The chance that the attraction will be mutual is only 18 per cent. Why is this so? Why does the one we want not always want us, and the one who wants us often seem unappealing to us? This phenomenon is called the "trap of the law of the social ladder", popularly known as the "endless singleness loop".

The endless singleness loop describes the phenomenon according to which we are more passionate about those who do not take much interest in us and, in contrast, show indifference toward those who are passionate about us. Apparently, there is no logic to this; it seems like a deliberate sabotaging of our chances for a relationship. But, again, evolution is to blame. We, like all other naturally social creatures, live in a social hierarchy and wish to mate with those who are equal to us or higher than us in that hierarchy. The reasoning goes that if someone is really into me, they probably belong to a league below me, which makes them less attractive. And if he's not particularly impressed with me, he's probably in a league above me, which is why he's more attractive. Our reptilian brain labels those who behave as if they are "hard to get" as being higher on the social ladder than us, while those who court us enthusiastically are marked down as being lower on the ladder.

Women are more likely to obey the law of rank. A man's overzealous courtship can turn a woman off, and the tough, unattainable macho man garners more success. More than once I've heard educated and high-achieving women say that they ended a relationship with a man because he was "too good". My friend Ronit, who is gifted with extraordinary honesty, says that she has to have the alpha man, the one who is hard to get and who is wanted by other women. To such types, she feels an animalistic sexual attraction, even though she knows that nothing good comes out of them in the end.

Well, do we control genes or do they control us? Judge for yourselves.

So, we've realized that the chances of finding "the one" are minimal and stand at 1:562 in England. When it comes to looking for a match, when should you stop searching? How many dates do you have to go on before you decide that you have found "the one"? To further refine this question, it is possible and indeed desirable to turn to the maths and treat this quandary as an optimization problem: what is the optimal number of dates to have before we decide that we have found "the one"? Dr Marianne Freiberger from the Faculty of Mathematics at the University of Cambridge used a formula for solving optimum problems developed in the 1960s for this purpose. The formula is not very complex, and we will not go into the details, but the result that Dr Freiberger reached was 37 per cent, meaning that after dating 37 per cent of the people we intend to date in our lifetime, we should marry the first one who comes along who is better than those who came before. There may be an element of risk in this, because perhaps someone better is waiting down the road, but in terms of risk management, optimization and maximization of probabilities, this is the best decision.

However, since we have no idea how many people we will meet in our entire lifetime, it is better to decide how long we intend to devote to finding a partner and calculate 37 per cent of that number. Suppose we intend to devote 21 years of our lives to finding a partner, from the age of 19 to the age of 40. If we consider 37 per cent of 21 years, the answer is 7.8 years. When we add this number to the age of 19, we reach 26.8. All of which would suggest that the first person we meet after reaching the age of 27 who we think is better and more suitable than anyone who came along before – he or she will be the one for us. That is the optimal strategy. Because of their biological clock, men can extend the age for finding a partner beyond the age of 40, which can give them a few more years. Nevertheless, it is interesting to note that the average age of marriage in the Western world today falls between 27 and 28 years. It turns out that this calculation takes place without our even being aware of it.

Love in the Digital Age

As we have seen, technology has upended all areas of our lives, including the world of courtship and marital love. A third of couples in the Western world today get to know each other through apps and websites. It is estimated that by 2040, 70 per cent of couples will have met each other in the digital space. On the one hand, in the entire history of mankind, single men and women have never had so many opportunities to meet new people. On the other, the experience of most surfers on dating sites is one of frustration and despair. They point to the chasm between people's profiles and the reality, the outright lies, the lack of seriousness and sudden disappearances (i.e., ghosting) – these are just some of the common experiences. In their banners and advertisements, dating platforms promise love, long-term relationships and even marriage, but a glance at their business model usually shows that the success of the platform doesn't depend on the number of successful matches, the percentage of marriages or the average length of the relationship, but on the length of time that users spend on the app. This is called the TOD model – "time on device". When their users spend more time on an app, that company's profits increase. Tragically, however, the more time a user spends on a platform, the less likely they are to bond with one person for the long term.

On the Tinder app, for example, there are 6 billion swipes to the right or left and 26 million matches per day. You swipe right for the people you want to get to know, and to the left for the ones you're not interested in. An average user logs onto Tinder four times a day and swipes an average of 120 times a day, a very long TOD, which also explains why the company's value is estimated at billions of dollars. But the important question is, is our brain built for this flood of information?

Never, in all the years of evolution, has a brain on Earth been exposed to so many sexual and emotional stimuli all at the same time. Before the advent of the digital age, in an average era in an average village, people of a reproductive age would know a limited number of potential partners from their village or from the neighbouring villages. Our brains are designed to handle a limited amount of data at one time. The big leap into the digital dating world requires the brain to absorb, filter and process a significant amount of data about many people all at once and then reach a quick decision. This creates a large cognitive load on the brain, which weakens the decision-making mechanisms operating in the prefrontal cortex, the area of rational thought. These processes consume a lot of energy and are seven times slower than the non-rational processes that occur in the primitive emotional brain. To cope with the data overload while browsing through many profiles, the primitive brain kicks in, quickly filters and eliminates, ruling out profiles first of all based on appearance, height, weight, age, social status and geographic location. The more profiles we browse, the more judgemental and critical we become and the faster we rule them out. Our criticism and negativity increase even more if we have already accumulated past disappointments or encountered major inconsistencies between people's profiles and the reality behind them.

Disappointing dating experiences are quite common in digital dating, where major discrepancies can exist between somebody's profile and the truth. This is because on dating sites most people lie most of the time. According to a study done in the Department of Psychology at the University of Berkeley, in which 1 million dating site profiles were examined, it was found that 81 per cent of the people in the profiles lied about their age, height and weight. Other studies have shown that women lie more about their age and weight and men lie more about their height, marital status and social standing. A third of people upload outdated photos to dating apps. As we have seen, cheating strategies for reproductive purposes are really nothing new in the evolutionary landscape. But this particular situation requires the brain to invest a lot of resources in detecting deception, which increases judgement and negativity and ultimately leads to frustration and despair.

So if we know that spending a long time on dating apps – and repeatedly checking if someone has swiped in our direction or sent us a message – causes cognitive overload and keeps us away from a stable relationship, why can't we stop logging on to these apps? The case of a good friend of mine sums it up perfectly. At the age of 35, Yael signed up (not for the first time) to an app and started going on dates with the aim of finding a partner. Most of the men didn't appeal to her, and her first few dates were not very successful. Then, one day, an interesting guy approached her, they corresponded, and after a while they went on a date. The date was nice and she had a good feeling about it. In the middle of the date, the guy went to the bathroom, and Yael took out her phone and absentmindedly opened the app to see what other messages she had received. She was so focused on the phone that she didn't notice the guy return to the table, walk behind her and see that she was answering messages from the website. There was an embarrassed pause and after that evening, he didn't make contact again. Yael was very upset. She called me and asked me to explain the meaning of this completely irrational behaviour of hers. She was interested in the guy, the date seemed to be going well, so why did she feel the urge to check whether there were other messages on the dating app?

This psychological phenomenon has a name, FOMO – fear of missing out – the fear of potentially missing something better. We don't allow ourselves to slow down, take our time with the person in front of us and really consider what they have to offer, if there are plenty more options out there, around the corner. Someone once said to me that it's similar to staying in a hotel and using a new towel after every shower, simply because there are so many new clean towels on the shelf in front of us. The FOMO phenomenon is much more common than it seems, because of the way the brain is structured, and it does a lot of damage to the ability of both men and women to connect and form long-term relationships. As mentioned, never in all the years of evolution have there been so many minds flooded with so much stimuli, so many opportunities and possibilities. Until we modern humans came on the scene, this inherited command and control centre of ours only had to function and make decisions under conditions of scarcity, such as dealing with a lack of food, a lack of breeding partners and a constant state of danger.

What happens when our brain buckles under a load of stimuli? In this instance, the brain activates its stress response. A stress response is a primitive survival mechanism whose role is to prepare the body and brain of an animal to deal with a challenging situation. The stress response causes inhibition of the prefrontal cortex, the area of rational thought that controls attention and concentration, and activates the irrational survival software of the ancient emotional brain – "fight or flight or freeze in place", with speed at the expense of accuracy.

In a stressful situation, there is no time for slow and reasoned processes; we have to make decisions quickly "from the gut", relying on our intuition.

This might be to run away ("flight") or to give up in advance and not make any decisions at all ("freeze in place"). When the emotional mind takes the reins in managing our love life, our anxieties are in charge. Our attention decreases, our ability to concentrate decreases, and our reluctance to take risks and disappointments increases: *Maybe something better is waiting for me? Maybe it won't work, I'm tired of being disappointed. What if he/she leaves me again?* And so the most important decisions in life are made hastily and irrationally and are biased toward negativity.

When you understand how our brains work, it's no surprise that technology has killed love. The brain is not an analytical supercomputer that, the more data we feed into it, the more comparisons it can make at breakneck speed to present us with the best choice. Our mind is an emotional machine that is operated by our emotional conditioning and biases, which were hardwired into our minds by the environment in which we grew up, and by the environment in which our ancestors survived. When this emotion machine encounters something it has never met before, it causes a system disruption.

An example of this kind of system disruption can be seen in the behaviour of Tinder users. We saw that the average Tinder user logs on to the app about 120 times a day. Tinder recently decided to limit its users to 100 right swipes daily. The reason for the restriction is that Tinder has noticed that there are quite a few users who swipe right not because they hope to get acquainted with somebody, but just to see if others want them. To these users they gave the name "indiscriminate narcissists". So has everyone become a narcissist, or is this related to the effect of technology on the emotional brain, which causes a relentless obsessive drive to open apps?

B F Skinner was a well-known American psychologist of the 1930s. Skinner, like Pavlov, was one of the forefathers of behaviourism. This systematic approach focuses on the study of visible human behaviour and the ways in which it can be shaped. Behaviourism studies how responses from the environment, be they positive or punishing, shape the behaviour of humans as they do that of other animals. Skinner was a radical behaviourist in that he believed the inner workings of the mind should be examined, too. He argued that mental states are physical states, and that they should therefore be studied in the same way that overt behaviour is studied.

In one of his famous experiments he built a box – now known as the "Skinner box" – that contains a light bulb, a food tray and a pedal. The box works so that when the light is on, a gentle press on the pedal releases a small amount of food into the food tray. Skinner experimented with a rat, a dog and a pigeon. All the animals learned the conditioning very quickly and pressed the pedal every time the light came on so that they could eat. After a while, when the animals realized that the food always came when the bulb was lit, they only pressed the pedal when they were hungry.

Then Skinner changed the rules and created a situation where sometimes pressing the pedal when the light came on led to food, but at other times no food was delivered even when the light was on. The animals entered a state of uncertainty and the results of the experiment became dramatic. Regardless of whether the light was on or off, the animals did not stop pressing the pedal until they reached a state of exhaustion; some even died from their exertions.

The explanation for this is that under conditions of inconsistent and uncertain positive reinforcement, there is a disruption of the reward system in the brain, which causes the activation of the stress response. The result is addictive obsessive-compulsive behaviour. The reward system in the emotional brain releases dopamine and creates a feeling of pleasure in response to certain stimuli. This system also creates links between different events that are related to positive reinforcements. However, a situation involving unexpected reinforcements or contradictory events disrupts the system and activates the stress response, which in turn triggers obsessive behaviour in order to produce certainty and try to take control of the situation.

In many respects, a mobile phone loaded with apps is a Skinner box for the 21st century. These apps offer unexpected and inconsistent positive reinforcements. Sometimes we open the app and there is positive reinforcement that causes pleasure: new messages, likes, swipes to the right in our direction, invitations to date, new profiles, a funny video and so forth. But sometimes we click and there's nothing interesting. And so we, like Skinner's wretched rats and pigeons and dogs, find ourselves obsessively and irrationally repeatedly logging on to apps and pressing the pedal endlessly, to the point of exhaustion and despair. The bad news is that today brain and behaviour researchers are complicit in the design of these apps, which capitalize on our human weaknesses so that we spend as much time as possible on them without pausing to consider the consequences on our mental state. In this distressed state of the brain, which is not built for such a load of stimuli, finding love and a long-term relationship becomes even more difficult.

The impact of technology on relationships can be seen in studies that compare relationships which originally started online with relationships that started in the real world. Professor Aditi Paul from the University of

Michigan, who studies the effects of technology on relationships, conducted a comparative study between the relationships of 4,000 couples who met on dating sites and who met IRL (i.e., in real life) in other ways. She found that couples who met online were three times more likely to divorce and 28 per cent more likely to break up in the first year. These couples were also less likely to get married in the first place and the quality of their relationship was lower than that of couples who met outside the network, through friends, family, work, and so on.

The explanation she offers for her findings is that both the means of communication and people's behaviour on digital platforms make it easier for them to end a relationship and move on to someone else. We are very social creatures and a romantic relationship is just one of the webs of relationships that make up our world. The better the relationship connects to the existing social fabric, the greater its chances of success. Technology creates new modes of communication in a space that challenges all social norms.

If so, what can we conclude from this – is it worthwhile or not to use technology for the purpose of finding a relationship and love? First, it is important to make the distinction between casual sex and a long-term commitment. The difference is huge, but the same platforms claim to provide both on demand. Click in the appropriate box if you are interested in a non-committed relationship, a committed relationship or a polyamorous relationship, and the application will create the match. At this point, Darwin would be laughing his socks off. How many applications will a man receive if he suggests that he is looking for a non-committed relationship, or a short-term romance, compared to a man who declares that he is "over the fooling around stage"? How would you label a woman who announces that she is only looking for casual sex versus a woman who declares that she is looking for someone to grow old with? We are a product of our biology and environment, living under social and evolutionary dictates. We can't really say what we want, and we are already so confused that we don't even know what we do want; so we say what we are expected to say and sometimes end up hurting ourselves and others. It is important to understand that we are very sexual creatures, the most sexual in the animal kingdom. We have sex out of social needs and not just for reproductive needs. The largest testicles in the animal kingdom relative to body size belong to the human male. Sex strengthens our social bonds and is important for our mental health. Sex for us is an existential drive, and long-term love is an added bonus. Looking for sex and long-term love on the same platform is like looking for a holiday cottage and a family home in the same place.

So, the first rule is to try to understand what we are really looking for at our stage of life, and also to understand the limitations of both dating sites and of humans. If your goal is to find a long-term relationship, you should reduce the use of apps that are mainly intended for casual sex.

The second rule is to connect with your emotional brain. What suits one person does not necessarily suit another. Do you feel that searching on dating sites does not benefit you, that it increases your frustrations and anxieties and causes you emotional instability? Do you react badly to disappointing dates, become suspicious and critical because of the many inconsistencies between what appears on dating profiles and the reality behind them, or take it to heart when people seem to vanish mid-sentence or after a date? If so, then this medium may not suit your emotional system and you should search outside the network, which will cause you less stress.

The third rule is to maintain a healthy balance. It is better to use apps as an additional means of dating and not as your main source. You should also limit the time you spend on the app to avoid obsession and behavioural addiction. It is advisable not to spend a lot of time endlessly scrolling through profiles so as not to increase your brain's judgemental, critical and negative bias. (The negativity bias is our tendency to lend more weight to the negative characteristics of a person than to their positive characteristics.) It is useful to focus your attention on a limited number of options so as not to increase the possibilities for distraction. Surveys show that most app interactions end after four messages. It is also advisable not to make a lot of phone calls or WhatsApp messages before a date, because when it comes to romance we have a tendency to idealize reality. We imagine an ideal partner based on their voice on the phone and the things he or she wrote, and this can end in disappointment during an actual face-to-face meeting. Rather than introduce this potential obstacle into a relationship before it has even got off the ground, it is better to meet as soon as possible or to talk in a video call – if possible, meet the speaker behind the voice early on in the process.

Another piece of advice is to limit the number of dates per week or per month so as not to cause your brain to overload and lower your attention span, which will lead to disappointment. A limited number of carefully selected dates will increase your chances of creating a long-term relationship. You shouldn't be fooled by the narcissistic need we all have to receive positive feedback about ourselves, our looks, our sexuality or our intellect, by multiplying your dates and conquests.

Last rule: do not go on dates with several people at the same time. Be empathetic both to your own mind and also to the people who want to get to know you. Processing too many encounters creates an overload on the emotional system, increases the anxiety of missing out (FOMO), reduces the ability to pay attention and will not allow you to create oxytocin and a real relationship with one person, because your brain will be so busy with comparative analysis.

Be Realistic About Your Options

The average age of marriage for women in the Western world is consistently on the rise. If we look at the records, we see that historically the average age of marriage for women remained more or less constant, at between 17 and 21, until it suddenly started to trend upwards, rising sharply in the 1990s to between 27 and 28. From the 2000s and onwards, it has even reached the age of 34 in Sweden and some other countries. From the moment the feminist revolution opened the doors to academia, the labour market and politics, women have been increasingly postponing the age of marriage. Generation Z women want to realize themselves in a way that their mothers and grandmothers couldn't even dream of. Today, in free-market economies, they go through higher education in greater percentages than men, advance quickly up the career ladder and try to postpone starting a family for as long as possible, all of which exacts a heavy toll.

The changes that human society and especially women have undergone in the last two centuries are enormous by any measure, but one thing remains exactly the same as it was 200 years, even 200,000 years ago: the reproductive age of women. Female fertility still starts at about age 12, drops sharply after age 35 and ends on average at age 40. The technological revolution has not changed the biology of reproduction at all. On the contrary, industrialization, overcrowding and technology have only caused a decrease in human fertility. The common myth sold to women – that 30 is the new 20 – is simply not true. From the age of 32, a woman's uterine fertility begins to decline and it does not seem that this is set to change any time in the near future. That's why if you're a woman who wants children, you should seriously dedicate your 20s to finding a partner, and not wait for a knight on a white charger to come galloping over the horizon.

Just as we devote energy and time to choosing a profession and managing our careers in rational ways, so we must do the same with our love life and choosing a committed partner. A career can be changed, as can a place of work and a place of residence, but we cannot easily swap the person who fathers our children for another – and if we wish to raise a family, the decisions we take about our long-term partner will impact our future quality of life, our happiness and the happiness of our children.

When we are looking to choose a partner for the long term, and in particular for raising a family, it is important to consider which qualities that person has that will remain relevant, such as emotional stability and security, parental and family abilities, and compatibility. In order to make rational decisions about relationships, we must regulate the messages that come from the ancient reptilian brain, which guides us to lend more weight to somebody's external appearance. Even if sometimes we don't get turned on immediately by someone and there is no attraction there at first sight, if we work on getting to know each other more deeply we will start to create experiences together; the oxytocin rises and with it come feelings of closeness, trust and even euphoria. The other person suddenly seems more attractive to us.

Give oxytocin a chance; don't dismiss it out of hand! Opposites may initially seem more attractive but, in the end, those with similarities are the ones who remain. All in all, it makes sense that over time we will get along better and have fewer disagreements with those who are more similar to us in our personality traits, in the way they solve problems, and in the type of family we would like to establish, which will often be similar to the families in which we grew up. Life is a journey full of challenges, changes and confrontations, and, on the whole, the laws of attraction are such that the more similar people are in their view of reality and in their approach to conflict resolution, the greater their chances will be of overcoming difficulties together.

CHAPTER 3
SAME-SEX LOVE AND ATTRACTION

Love is love is love. As far as the biological mechanisms of bonding, attachment and the role of the love hormones are concerned, there is no difference between two people of the same sex falling in love and two people of different sexes falling in love. The mechanisms are the same. The only difference in same-sex love lies in attraction.

The biology of love applies to all human beings regardless of their sexual orientation, with attraction being principally determined by signs of health and fertility among the same species. Handsome is drawn to beautiful and beaus to belles; and with some couples this just happens to take place within the same gender. Even in a same-sex relationship, it is sometimes possible to see an attraction to male or female characteristics within the couple, which has been called the butch-femme dichotomy and relates to the draw of the male to the female – the dance between testosterone and oestrogen. The desire for connection between males and females is probably a global characteristic of life on Earth.

In this book, I deal at length with the differences between the sexes – between the female brain and the male brain, and between the feelings and needs of both sexes, some of which are biological and others of which are shaped by education and society. I believe that this knowledge can contribute to increasing empathy between the sexes. Understanding our differences should lead to a more effective resolution of relationship conflicts and help to preserve committed relationships over time. For me, the references in this book to the differences between men and women actually refer first and foremost to the differences between male and female, between testosterone and oestrogen, regardless of the specific reproductive system a person has or their sexual orientation – and this approach can be applied to both same-sex love and bisexual love.

The Biology of Sexual Orientation

What are the biological factors that affect our sexual orientation and sexual identity, attracting some boys and girls to the same sex as themselves? The science, like everything else related to humans, is complex. There are few clear answers to the question of which biological factors determine sexual attraction in humans. Indeed, there aren't many other topics in human biology that are quite as complex and politically charged as that of sexual orientation and identity, so scientists tend to shy away from getting to the heart of the matter.

Nevertheless, a growing body of research on the subject indicates that sexual orientation and identity have a biological basis, and that they originate from biological factors and not from lifestyle choices. In every human society that has been studied, between 2 and 10 per cent of the population have same-sex orientation. Similar numbers are also found in the rest of the animal kingdom. Homosexual behaviour has been observed in about 1,500 species of animals. The bonobo, known too as the pygmy chimpanzee, is genetically closest to us in the animal kingdom, and also the most bisexual animal. Among the lions, probably to ensure loyalty in the group, there are males who mate with other males and thus strengthen the bonds between them. Among ducks and geese, which form monogamous pairs, 4 to 5 per cent of pairs are same-sex. The same goes for penguins. In 2019, a pair of homosexual penguins in a zoo in the Netherlands were so eager to raise offspring that they stole an egg from a pair of heterosexual penguins and took care of it. Courtship and cohabitation among members of the same species have also been observed among dolphins. In giraffes, a high percentage of homosexual interactions is found between males, especially after attacks, and a much lower percentage of such interactions is found between females. In a population of squid, there is a small percentage of the males that look like females, smaller and colourless. They join the harem of a large alpha male squid, who is sure they are females and mates with them. Fourteen per cent of seagulls have lesbian pairings. Among black swans in Australia, 6 per cent of pairs are exclusively male. Eight per cent of male sheep are attracted to male partners only.

What is the Evolutionary Advantage of Homosexuality?

Since same-sex behaviour is very common throughout the animal kingdom, there is a hypothesis that it offers a survival advantage, even though – from a purely Darwinian evolutionary perspective – homosexuality does not appear to advance the interests of the selfish gene, since it is not the best way for an individual to pass on his or her genetic material to the next generation. So what, then, is the advantage of homosexuality for genes? The answer is that the survival advantage lies not only at the level of the individual's own selfish genes but at the level of the genetic pool of the group or tribe.

This theory holds that homosexual behaviour strengthens the social bonds between the individuals in a group, reduces competitiveness and thus promotes the survival of the group as a whole. Same-sex behaviour increases group oxytocin through courtship and sexual contact, lowers testosterone levels and aggression, and consequently also lowers cortisol/stress levels within the entire group. This, in turn, strengthens the social ties in the group and thus helps to increase the support available for raising offspring. Moreover, homosexuality among males reduces the competition between males for females, thereby reducing violence between the males in the group. So, to sum up, a group that has homosexual individuals will transfer more of its genes to the next generation compared to a group that has none.

You may have already come across the idea of a group acting like a super-organism in which the individuals collectively promote the genes of the group and do not necessarily reproduce by themselves. For example, ants and bees are species wherein only the queen passes her genes on to future generations and all the other individuals specialize in different roles to help the group effort. The evolutionary success of these social species is among the most impressive in the animal kingdom.

Another evolutionary theory, which tries to explain why homosexuality has not disappeared from the gene pool, is called the "fertile female" hypothesis. A study undertaken in Italy showed that the daughters of families that include homosexual men have 1.3 times more children on average than the daughters of families with only heterosexual men. One possible explanation for this is that the daughters of homosexual men's families have the trait of homosexuality and that this causes them to have more children at an earlier time of life, perhaps as a compensatory mechanism for a lack of children from their homosexual family members. Another explanation is that the support and assistance that homosexual family members give to the daughters of their family make it easier for them to have more children.

At this point in time, all theories regarding the evolutionary advantages that homosexuality offers various species on Earth are just educated guesses. Extensive genetic studies are needed among different populations of humans and different animal groups to confirm them.

Is Sexual Orientation Genetic?

To answer the question of whether sexual orientation is genetic, and, if so, which genes are responsible for it, studies were done on identical twins. In these studies, it was found that the chance of a male twin being homosexual if his twin brother was homosexual was 20 per cent. The chance of homosexuality in the general human population ranges from 2 to 10 per cent. That is, a homosexual identical twin brother increases the chance of his twin brother being homosexual by two to ten times.

The first attempt to identify the "gay gene" occurred in 1993 when molecular genetics professor Dean Hamer and his colleagues from the National Institutes of Health (NIH) in the United States examined the genomes of 38 homosexual identical twins compared to the genomes of heterosexual twins. Hamer and his colleagues characterized a specific region in the genome on the X chromosome, called the Xq28 region, which they saw in the genomes of the homosexual twins but not in the genomes of the heterosexuals.

Six years later, another study was carried out by Professor John Bailey and his colleagues at the University of Cambridge in the USA, this time on 400 pairs of homosexual male twins. The researchers found that the Xq28 region is indeed associated with sexual preference in men. They found another region on chromosome 8, the 8q12 region, which appeared more often in the homosexual brothers. In 2017, they repeated the experiment using a wider analysis of the genomes of 1,077 homosexual men compared to the genomes of 1,231 heterosexual men, and found additional regions associated with same-sex preference.

The largest study carried out to date in an attempt to decipher the genetics of sexual preference involved over half a million genomes of men with a homosexual sexual orientation. The study discovered five regions in the genome – genetic markers – that are associated with sexual preference. However, the researchers were unable to use any of these genetic markers to predict an individual's sexual orientation based on a random genome presented to them. The study, published in 2019 in the journal *Science* and carried out by researchers from MIT, Harvard and Cambridge, supported the findings from previous research, which included a smaller number of subjects, and confirmed the hypothesis of many scientists: that while sexual orientation has a genetic component, there is no single gene that influences this tendency. Actually, there is no "pride gene", a gene responsible for homosexuality. Geneticist research leader Dr Andrea Gana from the Broad

Institute at MIT estimates that while up to 25 per cent of same-sex attraction can be explained by genetics, the rest may be down to environmental factors.

Environment and the "Big Brother Effect"

One finding, which has been repeated across several studies, is that a man's chance of being homosexual increases with each adult male sibling he has in the family. The discovery of this phenomenon, nicknamed "the big brother effect", arose from research carried out over two decades, which analysed statistical data and showed that the existence of grownup biological older brothers, but not sisters, increase the likelihood of their younger male sibling being homosexual. The studies found that the chance increases by 33 per cent with each adult male sibling in the family. (That is, if the probability of homosexuality in the general population is 2 to 10 per cent, each adult sibling increases this by 33 per cent.)

In 1996, the Canadian psychologist Professor Anthony Bogaert and his colleague Ray Blanchard built on findings from the late 1950s that indicated homosexual men tend to have a greater number of older siblings, and published research that argued homosexuality is more common in those men who specifically have older brothers. The researchers also argued that the effect is not related to environmental factors but to biological factors. Studies compared the likelihood of young boys being homosexual in families with biological siblings, with families containing non-biological siblings (i.e., not from the same parents), and found the likelihood of homosexuality in the younger boys was found to be high only when the siblings were biological.

Researchers then replicated Bogaert's study among Indonesian men. They examined data from 116 Indonesian homosexual men and 62 heterosexual men, and also found that the homosexual men were more likely to have older male siblings than heterosexual men were.

In 2006, Bogaert and his colleagues examined data from 3,146 Canadian homosexual men and concluded that the influence of the "older brother effect" on the sexuality of a younger son was also linked to another factor: left-handedness or right-handedness. They found that the effect of older male siblings on the likelihood of homosexuality occurred only in right-handed men and not in left-handed men. Left-handedness develops in the embryonic stages; therefore it can be assumed that certain biological processes which occur in the embryonic stages cause an increase in the likelihood of homosexuality in those right-handed embryos with older brothers.

In 2017, the process responsible for the "big brother effect" was pinpointed when a group of researchers from Brock University and Harvard confirmed findings that indicate sexual orientation in men is probably determined in the womb. In the largest laboratory experiment of its kind to involve the mothers of gay men, the following groups were tested:

- 72 mothers of heterosexual men
- 31 mothers of gay men without older brothers
- 23 mothers of gay men with older brothers
- 16 childless women
- a control group of 12 men

The researchers tested the reactions of the immune system and antibodies of all the women to two proteins that are found only in men and which appear in the brain of the male foetus. They discovered that the mothers of the homosexual men, especially the mothers of gay men with older brothers, had higher levels of these antibodies than all the other groups of women and the control group. The researchers believe that during the first pregnancy or immediately after the birth of the first son, in some women, the immune system begins to recognize the male proteins and develops an immune response (antibodies) against them. With each additional birth of a son, the ever-increasing levels of these antibodies to combat the proteins in the male foetal brain affect the brain development of the boys born later. The hypothesis is that this is the mechanism responsible for the "big brother effect".

The "big brother effect", in which the number of boys born to a mother affects the sexual orientation of her younger sons, strengthens the evolutionary arguments for homosexuality reducing competition and conflicts between the males in the pack over females and thereby increasing social cohesion. Also, among some other animals, the ratio between the number of males and the number of females in an environment has an effect on the sexual orientation and identity of the individuals that occupy it. For example, in certain fish species, when all the males in a group are killed, one of the females then becomes a male. Such sex changes also happen in the opposite scenario, where the females disappear and one of the males becomes a female. The mechanism responsible for this sex change in mid-life is epigenetic: a change in the presentation of genes through stimulation from the environment. (Epigenetic changes are acquired chemical changes that occur in the genes in response to environmental stimuli. The stimuli from the environment cause a change in the way the DNA is organized and subsequently a change in genetic appearance; this means that the epigenetic change acts rather like an on–off switch for the genes, which is activated in response to signals from the environment.) In some species of fish, reptiles and birds, the sex of the embryo can be affected by temperature changes or other changes in the environment.

Exposure to Testosterone in Utero

There are other factors in the mother's womb that affect the sexual orientation and identity of the developing foetus. There are studies that show how early exposure of the foetus to high levels of hormones such as testosterone affects sexual orientation in adulthood. Exposure to testosterone during the embryonic stage of development influences the development of the brain and body. The "finger ratio" in the hand, for example, is believed to be one of the things that is affected by exposure to testosterone in utero. On average, the higher the foetus's exposure to testosterone, the smaller the ratio between the length of the index finger and the ring finger. That is, the index finger in men is usually shorter than the ring finger, but the index finger in women is usually longer than the ring finger. This finger ratio can also hint at sexual orientation. Studies have found that in homosexual men there is a greater chance that the index finger will be longer than the ring finger, as in heterosexual women. Among lesbian women, it was found that there is a higher chance that the index finger will be shorter than the ring finger, as in heterosexual men.

Testosterone also affects spatial perception. On average, men do better at spatial vision tasks, such as matching patterns and angles, than women. However, the evidence suggests that homosexual men tend to be less successful than heterosexual men in these tasks, while lesbian women are often more successful in them than heterosexual women.

Other studies show that homosexual men are 31 per cent more likely to be left-handed than heterosexual men, while lesbian women are 91 per cent more likely to be left-handed. Homosexual men are 15 per cent more likely to have anti-clockwise hair whorls (parietal whorls), because the gene that determines the direction of hair growth is linked to left-handedness and sexual orientation. Left-handedness was also found to be related to testosterone levels early in development.

But testosterone doesn't explain everything. Studies show that female foetuses are also exposed to small levels of testosterone, which is secreted from their adrenal gland, from the placenta and from the mother's hormonal system. At key points after fertilization, male and female embryos are exposed to similar levels of testosterone. The levels can even be higher than normal in female foetuses, and lower than normal in male foetuses without any effect on the structure of the reproductive system or the structure of the brain. Studies also reveal that male foetuses and female foetuses react differently to hormones in their environment. Their sensitivity to hormones remains different, even while a particular hormone level is temporarily higher.

Researchers from the University of California at Santa Barbara believe that the difference in the sensitivity of male and female foetuses to sex hormones is the result of epigenetic changes. When the foetus develops in its mother's womb, certain sex-related genes are turned on and off by an epigenetic process, in response to different levels of the sex hormones in the womb, which are secreted by both the foetus and the mother. This hormonal "struggle" affords a certain advantage to the foetus by keeping the development of the male or female on track, even during sharp and sudden increases in the levels of hormones in the womb, either on the part of the mother or on the part of the foetus itself.

At key points during the development of the foetus, epigenetic changes in the pathways that testosterone uses to exert its effects can reduce or increase sensitivity to the hormone and thus change its effect on the body of the foetus and influence the design of the brain. According to a ground-breaking study by the Californian researchers, published in 2012, if these epigenetic changes continue once the baby is born and goes on to have its own children, some of its offspring may be homosexual. The leader of the research, the evolutionary geneticist Professor William Rice, believes there is a reason why homosexuality does not disappear over the generations, and that reason is epigenetics.

Epigenetic influences are probably the missing piece in the puzzle of the biology of sexual orientation. To deepen our understanding of the epigenetic mechanisms that influence sexual orientation, geneticist Eric Vilain and his colleagues from the University of California looked for epigenetic markers on the genomes of homosexual men. (As mentioned, epigenetic markers are chemical changes in DNA that affect gene expression.) The researchers collected DNA from 37 pairs of identical twins in which one of the twins was homosexual, and from 10 pairs of identical twins who were both homosexual. Then they scanned the epigenome of the twins. The epigenome is the sum of all the epigenetic markers in the genome, all the chemical changes in the DNA of the genome. The researchers found five epigenetic markers that were shared by all the homosexual twin brothers and which were not found in the heterosexual twin brothers. One marker was found on a gene related to brain development, a second marker was found on a gene related to the immune system, and the others appeared in areas not related to the expression of any gene. Relying on these five markers alone, the researchers developed an algorithm that was able to predict with 67 per cent accuracy the sexual orientation of a random person, based on the five markers in the epigenome.

It is important to say at this point there are limitations to this study. Firstly, the sample was not large enough to draw clear conclusions regarding the complex epigenetics of sexual orientation. Secondly, epigenetic markers are different in cells found in different tissues in the body, and while it is likely that those present in the cells of the brain have the greatest relevance to sexual preference, those cells were not tested in the study.

It is not surprising that epigenetics has a role in shaping sexual orientation, although there is still no information about the specific environmental factors that are associated with these markers and the relevant genes affected by them. It can be assumed that with further developments in the relatively new and fascinating field of epigenetics, it will be possible to understand more in the future about the complicated connections between environmental factors and the shaping of sexual orientation.

Asexuality

Alfred Kinsey was one of the first researchers in the field of human sexual behaviour. In the mid-20th century, the American biologist created a scale of sexual orientation between 0 and 6, ranging from heterosexuality to homosexuality, which came to be known as the Kinsey scale. Alongside this, he created a category he called "X", for those subjects "lacking relationships or socio-sexual connections". Today, this is the category that represents asexuals. It is estimated that 1 per cent of the population define themselves as asexual. They do not experience sexual attraction or sexual arousal, and do not feel the need to experience orgasm with another person. It's not a choice. This is their authentic, natural feeling.

One of the first known asexuals in history could be Isaac Newton, who was celibate until the end of his life and according to speculation fits into this grouping. Due to his inability to connect with people, some speculate that he can also be defined as being on the autism spectrum (Asperger syndrome). Is there a connection between these two conditions? There is evidence to suggest that some individuals who self-identify as asexual have also been officially diagnosed with autism disorder, which is typically characterized by difficulties in social interaction and communication. In addition, the literature shows that asexuality and lack of sexual attraction, or low sexual interest, are more common in people with autism spectrum disorder compared to the general population. However, not enough in-depth studies have been conducted on the relationship between autism and asexuality.

To sum up, the biological mechanisms of sexual orientation are complex and research on the subject is still in its infancy. Many more studies are needed involving both whole populations and individuals, and covering genetics, epigenetics and research into the hormones that influence sexual orientation and identity in humans and animals. However, what is clear is that same-sex attraction is one of the natural and most common phenomena on the planet and offers evolutionary survival advantages to many different groups of animals, including humans.

CHAPTER 4
FALLING IN LOVE

The word "love" comes from the Sanskrit *lobhayati*, "to make crazy". In this chapter we will discover how certain "love drugs" do indeed make us crazy at the beginning of a relationship – the "falling in love" phase. So let's dive into what starts to happen just after that first kiss, right after 50 million bacteria have passed from mouth to mouth and chorused, "Yes!" Now we are primed and ready to flood our brains with serious doses of love drugs, substances that will blow our heads off – and all that implies. Welcome to the roller coaster of falling in love!

During the falling in love phase, when we are with a new partner for the first time, our brain is drenched with the best substances a brain can receive, which are released during touching, caressing, kissing, soft massages and then at really high levels during sex.

It starts during the kiss, when the love hormone, oxytocin, is released from the brain into the bloodstream and saliva, and stimulates the vagus nerve, also known as the social nerve. At this moment you may feel a magical vibration, as if electricity is passing along your spinal cord to your lower back, lighting up your genitals and bringing them to life. We feel the sparks and heat rising from the genitals – wetness in the vagina, the erection of the penis, all the product of the effects of oxytocin, which is responsible for our sexual behaviour, the hormone of desire and orgasms. It's no coincidence that many people decide whether "this is it" or not based on a kiss.

When a male mouse is injected with oxytocin into his lower back, directly into the vagus nerve, an erection is immediately triggered. When oxytocin is injected into a female mouse's lower back, into the vagus nerve, she immediately raises her pelvis and lifts her bottom; this position is called lordosis and facilitates the penetration of the penis into the vagina. Lifting the pelvis in females is a transmitter of sexual motivation and oestrus for males. When we hear felines howling at night while on heat, they perform the lordosis position, raising the pelvis, and the tomcats are understandably beside themselves with excitement.

The instinct for the lordosis position, the lifting of the pelvis and the sexual message this broadcasts to the environment, still exists within us. This is why women in the Victorian period wore dresses that highlighted the rear and gave them the appearance of prominent, impressive lifted bottoms. These lordosis dresses were designed in this way to produce a more attractive and sexy look. The sexiness inherent in the lordosis position is also the reason why many women today are willing to pay the high price of orthopaedic injury to the back and legs caused by high heels. The high heel stiffens the back and creates a lordosis curve, which transmits a very sexually attractive message. It's no coincidence that in porn movies women often wear excessively high and thin heels.

Let's get back to that kiss. Our genitals are now stimulated by the oxytocin that is released during kissing and cuddling. We can feel the butterflies in our stomach, another sure sign that we are excited by the abundance of hormones flowing. Next, testosterone, the sex drive hormone, is called to attention by the multitude of smells and pheromones in the air and is released directly from the testicles into the bloodstream of the man and from the ovaries into the blood circulation of the woman. Testosterone produces sex drive, desire, libido and life energy.

At this stage, the old limbic emotional brain goes wild and demands orgasm (dopamine) *now*, while the evolutionary newer prefrontal cortex tries to control the situation and regulate behaviour. The fight between them begins: *Do I really want to do this? Is it right for me at this point? What will my parents/friends/family say? What will he/she think of me? Do I look good? Will I live up to expectations?* All those demons are created in our head. The more testosterone is released, the weaker our self-control will be, because testosterone inhibits the activity of the frontal lobe.

Brain scans have also shown that the frontal lobe in men turns off faster than in women during sexual activity. In women, the frontal lobe switches off only at the moment of orgasm itself. The evolutionary logic of the genes is clear: for the male, take advantage of every opportunity to reproduce, don't think twice, and spread your seed everywhere; for the female, you may have to invest all your energy in a little baby that will be created this magical evening, so think about all the consequences and don't be reckless! For most women, a whole heap of social-psychological-cultural dictates created by male-dominated societies are also piled on top of their evolutionary wiring.

A Question of Self-Control

The question nevertheless arises, if oxytocin is the hormone that produces all our social relationships and also acts on our genitals and results in sexual arousal, why doesn't the sexual urge arise in all our social relationships, such as with our friends and our work colleagues and even within the family? Well, arousal of the genitals can occur in any social situation under the influence of oxytocin, but this is when the frontal lobe, which suppresses sexual behaviour, enters the picture and exercises its judgement. If the situation is not appropriate according to the social norms of the society we live in, the frontal lobe will suppress our sexual arousal. This is why oxytocin is also called the context-dependent hormone. In any enjoyable social situation, the emotional brain (that is, the limbic brain) will release oxytocin, which in turn induces feelings of trust, closeness, ease and relaxation. However, the frontal lobe is the one in charge of the range of feelings that will be generated, and controls our behaviour according to social dictates and our own conscience and morality.

In situations when a person's frontal lobe is damaged, such as in some cases involving mental disability, it can be possible to see the difficulty experienced by that individual in suppressing their sexual arousal in social situations; and it may arise in inappropriate circumstances, for example in front of a caregiver for whom the person with the disability feels a strong feeling of love and closeness.

During adolescence, generally understood as occurring between the ages of 11 and 27 – when a young person's frontal lobe is still maturing – it can similarly be more difficult to exercise judgement and control behaviour, especially in the context of oxytocin and sexuality. But as each and every one of us will testify, this also happens long after the age of 27! Under sexual stimulation and the influence of oxytocin, our judgement and decision-making processes are impaired – and this is because of the structure of the brain. If you were to look at a cross-section of the brain, you would notice how the neural pathways that carry the stimuli from the environment (received through smell, taste, sound, touch and licking) to the emotional brain (the limbic brain) are much wider than the neural pathways that transmit the controlling and regulating stimuli from the frontal lobe to the emotional brain. In other words, there is a structural difficulty in regulating the emotional brain and controlling our emotion-based behaviour, especially when the intensity of environmental stimuli is heightened, as during sexual stimulation.

The characteristics of self-control are, of course, dependent on our society and culture. We humans are very social creatures, leaders of the animal kingdom in the amount of oxytocin we produce, which is probably why we are also the most sexual creatures in the animal kingdom. As previously mentioned, we use sex not only for reproductive purposes but for our social needs. We use sex and contact for social formation and the enrichment of our social connections. As mentioned, we are not the only ones to do this in the animal kingdom: bonobo apes, or pygmy chimpanzees, live in a matriarchal society that wants peace, sex and love, and they, like us, make love not only for reproductive purposes but for social reasons.

Sex and touch strengthen our social bonds and calm us down. Human societies today are very different from those in the past, in terms of their compliance with rules and restrictions on sexual–social behaviour. Rules, restrictions, norms, codes and overt and covert messages are absorbed and wired into the frontal lobe of every newborn baby in every society and in every era. They are reinforced through their parents or caregivers, family members, school, peer groups, country and culture. This wiring will accompany the baby for the rest of its life and will influence all its decision-making processes. As the baby grows into adult life, it will continue to inform that individual day by day and hour by hour, in a variety of social situations, about the potential long-term consequences of every decision originating in the emotional brain. However, as the emotional brain works seven times faster than the frontal lobe and receives a huge amount of stimuli from the environment, the bad news is that in 90 per cent of these battles, the emotional brain will win, and for a significant part of our lives we will be kept busy with damage limitation.

Just how difficult the struggle between the emotional and the rational systems in our brains is, especially in men, can be seen if we take a moment to consider the scale of domestic sexual abuse and sexual harassment in the workplace. The reason why men do more harm results from the effects of testosterone on the brain, which increases sex drive while simultaneously inhibiting the action of the frontal lobe, the lobe of judgement. When a heterosexual man is in the presence of a woman, and certainly during courtship, his testosterone level increases even more. Testosterone is the reason that boys and young men are more prone to impaired judgement than older men over the age of 60. A man's testosterone level does not remain the same throughout his life, but peaks at puberty, around the age of 15, and when he passes the age of 55 the level drops to about a fifth of the amount he had as a young man.

Studies have found higher than average levels of testosterone among rapists, sex offenders and murderers serving prison sentences. It is important to note that not every man with high testosterone is prone to crime and there are indeed quite a few men with medium and low levels of testosterone who are languishing in prison because of sex-related crimes. However, it is also clear that in castrated animals, once the testicles – which manufacture testosterone – have been removed, there is a decrease in their aggression and sex drive. In a study that examined the effects of testosterone in a group of men who were given a weekly dose of over 600mg of the hormone, it was found that many of them developed mental disorders characterized by excessive self-confidence, impulsiveness, making ill-judged actions, wasting money, excessive sexual activity, uncontrolled self-talk and aggression.

Sex, Drugs and . . . Love?

From the point of view of evolution, sexual activity is the main reason for our existence in the world. That's why our brains are programmed by our genes to produce the most pleasurable and rewarding bursts of neurochemicals at a very specific time – during sex. These chemicals, which produce a wide range of enjoyable, relaxing and beneficial pleasurable sensations, are released during sexual activity, spurring us on to experience more and more such magical moments and focus on passing our genes to the next generation, especially while we are fertile.

Here are the chemicals – or drugs, if you will – of sex:

1. The happiness drugs – the endorphins

Natural opioid-like chemicals – the body's natural morphine – are released from the brain, relieving pain and creating a good feeling, even euphoria. The endorphins are part of the brain's reward system and are released during sexual activity, during dangerous or strenuous physical activity such as running, while hugging children, when listening to music, when we dance and while laughing, for example. Endorphins are part of the set of survival chemicals and stimulate us into actions that support our survival, such as running away, hiding, mating and socializing. It is the endorphins that are responsible for the wonderful feelings enjoyed by those who perform difficult, dangerous and adrenaline-charged activities. They are released immediately after frightening and daring performances, whether sports or sex. Since endorphins are part of the brain's reward system, they can be addictive.

2. The stimulant – phenethylamine (PEA)

Phenethylamine is an amino acid that occurs naturally in the brain and is similar in its activity to amphetamines such as Ritalin. Phenethylamine is a stimulating psychoactive chemical that is secreted during sex and makes us feel like we are on top of the world – euphoric, energetic and able to stay up all night talking to our beloved. It is the substance that drives our infatuation with, and excitement at, being with our partner. It is also found in chocolate, which is why chocolate lifts the mood, and it is released during vigorous physical activities such as skydiving. Perhaps this is why falling in love sometimes feels like taking an exciting leap!

3. The elixir of life – testosterone

This is an anabolic sex hormone that builds muscle and tissue and is essential for both men and women. It is formed from cholesterol in the testicles of men and the ovaries of women. Testosterone is responsible for the sex drive and the libido in all of us, and in men it causes the creation of sperm. Testosterone greatly affects our emotional state and has a strong influence on the limbic brain. It elevates the mood, increases energy levels, vitality and motivation, and improves memory. A natural decrease in testosterone over the years is accompanied by a decrease in sex drive and an increase in feelings of despondency and lack of motivation. Testosterone increases during sports, especially in members of the winning side during competitive games. It also increases when we eat meat, when we are in the company of attractive people whom we find sexually appealing, during masturbation, while watching porn and, of course, most of all during sex.

During the day, the level of testosterone in the blood changes and it reaches its peak in men in the early morning upon waking, and in women at eight in the evening. That's why men usually want, initiate and respond better to sex in the morning, while women show more interest in the evening. A woman's testosterone levels fluctuate during her menstrual cycle; during ovulation there is an increase that leads to a heightened sex drive. In men and women, stress causes a decrease in testosterone, since the stress hormones, cortisol and adrenaline, suppress the secretion of hormones from the adrenal gland that in turn stimulates the secretion of testosterone. Therefore, stress causes a decrease in the sex drive of both men and women. Some men take testosterone pills or injections after the age of 55, and today a testosterone gel is available for women who suffer from a decrease in libido, to be applied to the skin before sexual activity.

4. The uplifting drug – serotonin

This is a neurochemical from the monoamine family (like dopamine and adrenaline) and plays a key role in creating pleasant feelings and preventing depression. During and after orgasm, high levels of serotonin are secreted, causing feelings of elation, self-confidence and joy. It is the hormone responsible for the feeling of conquest and the pleasure of falling under the spell of our partner as more orgasms are experienced together.

Serotonin is produced and stored in the intestinal cells. It is formed from tryptophan, which is the rarest amino acid in nature and is found in eggs, nuts and dairy products – all of which increase serotonin production. Sunlight also helps produce serotonin, so go outdoors and walk in nature to boost your levels. And if you do this with your partner, your relationship will strengthen.

New research shows that bacteria in the intestines stimulate cells to produce serotonin and thus affect our moods. The intestines are networked with neural pathways, and these nerves contain more than 500 million neurons, on which there are receptors for serotonin and other chemicals connected to the emotions. So it's no surprise that when we are head over heels in love we feel butterflies in our stomach: these are serotonin butterflies.

If our body lacks serotonin production, there follows an increase in depression and anxiety. Anti-anxiety drugs such as Ciprofloxacin and Prozac work on the brain by preventing the breakdown of serotonin in synapses (the connections between brain cells) and leaving it there longer. Studies show that having sex regularly reduces the risk of developing depression, since sexual activity produces serotonin. People who are sexually active are less likely to develop depression and more likely to have a more positive self-image and a stronger immune system. Therefore, with or without a permanent relationship, it is important to maintain a healthy level of sexual activity, with frequent masturbation and multiple orgasms for the brain. More orgasms, less Ciprofloxacin. In our stress-saturated digital age, there has been a corresponding decrease in sex drive, which leads to less intercourse, a decrease in serotonin production, an increase in depression, and a decrease in sex drive . . . it's a downward spiral.

5. The drug of pleasure and motivation – dopamine

Dopamine, as previously mentioned, is a central neurochemical in the brain. It is the reason we get up every morning and stir ourselves into action. Chemically, life itself is a constant search for small moments of pleasure – those moments when dopamine feeds straight into the pleasure and reward system of the emotional brain.

Dopamine is the reserve currency of the reward system. Therefore, any behaviour that stimulates the secretion of dopamine will encourage us to repeat it and even become addicted to it in certain situations. Eating is a behaviour that triggers dopamine, especially something tasty. Further down the scale, social connection, appreciation from those around us, high social status and control over others also lead to small doses of dopamine. The behaviour that evokes the highest level of dopamine of all is sex. The peak of dopamine secretion, the peak of reward, in any living being occurs during orgasm. That's what we're here for and that's what we'll be rewarded for. The genes, the programmers of our biological systems, drip drops of pleasure on us when we successfully carry out our tasks here – i.e., orgasms.

Thanks to the high level of dopamine released during orgasm, the more sexual activity between partners and the more orgasms experienced, the more a connection is formed in their minds between everything related to the partner (sight, sound, touch, smell) and pleasure. The ringing of the phone heralding the lover's voice triggers the release of dopamine and the pleasure of anticipation. The anticipation of the partner, the touch, the caress and the expected orgasm may be even more pleasurable than the moment itself. Because dopamine is such a powerful motivator, many of us will likely find ourselves searching for a partner and longing for love at some stage in our lives.

Any behaviour that triggers a significant release of dopamine and a strong stimulation of the reward system can give rise to addictive–compulsive behaviours to obtain pleasure. The more a person suffers from emotional barriers, depression or past traumas, the greater their risk of addiction. Drugs such as cocaine and heroin are highly addictive because they act on the dopamine system, and dopamine is also the reason people may become addicted to sex, porn and even to a partner and love. Another feature of the dopamine system in humans – and one of its most disappointing features – is that anything that becomes monotonous bores us over time. The same food, the same TV, the same friends, and to a greater extent sex with the same person, all bore us over time. (The sexual saturation effect, known as the Coolidge effect, and its impact on longer-lasting relationships over time will be discussed in chapter 6.)

6. Love drugs – oxytocin and vasopressin

The last drug to be released from the brain during orgasm to complete the experience and strengthen the bond is the aforementioned oxytocin, the brain's natural "ecstasy" (as in the psychoactive drug MDMA). When oxytocin is released, it immediately boosts the release of dopamine and serotonin, which is what makes love so rewarding and pleasurable. During orgasm, childbirth or breastfeeding, oxytocin acts on the muscles of the reproductive organs and causes them to contract. During the orgasm, it produces the orgasm contractions themselves – three seconds of contractions of the vagina, the muscles of the uterus and the anus in the woman, and of the spermatic cord, the prostate gland, the muscles around the penis and the anus in the man.

In addition, the more you produce this love hormone, the more you cuddle, touch, orgasm or even use a synthetic oxytocin inhaler, the tighter the relationship between you and your partner becomes. In a study in Germany, 29 couples were given a dose of synthetic oxytocin from an inhaler before intercourse. The couples, especially the men, reported more intense orgasms and a desire to curl up and cuddle after the orgasm. The women reported that they felt they were better able to share their sexual desires with their partner and show empathy.

In the real world, outside the lab, the same feelings of closeness, empathy and heightened pleasure arise when having sex with a partner we love and with whom we have a prior acquaintance, compared to having sex with a stranger. The difference lies in the high amount of oxytocin in the blood with partners we know and love, compared to a lower amount with a person we do not know.

As we have seen, both women and men secrete oxytocin, but in men, there is the release of another hormone during orgasm from the oxytocin family called vasopressin. Vasopressin is the male version of oxytocin. Oxytocin is a short protein made up of nine amino acids, which are the building blocks that make up every protein, and vasopressin differs in one amino acid out of the nine. In males, vasopressin causes a feeling of loyalty and a desire to protect their partner and offspring. It is secreted at a high level during orgasm and also when the male, especially the monogamous male, is near his mate and offspring.

In a study done at the National Institute of Mental Health in the USA, researchers injected vasopressin into socially monogamous American male prairie voles and were surprised to find that even when the males were in a cage with a sterilized female, which theoretically should not have aroused any sexual desire in them, they showed an affectionate attitude toward her, protecting her from strangers and becoming very territorial. Even when they were presented with other females, most of the male prairie voles preferred to return to the partner with whom they had "fallen in love" under the auspices of vasopressin. A similar reaction was also obtained in female prairie voles who received oxytocin and bonded with the male who was with them during the injection. As with the male voles, and also with us humans, the secret of long-term love and attachment lies in sexual activity and orgasms. The more we have sex with the same partner, and the more orgasms we experience, which act like injections of oxytocin and vasopressin directly into the brain, the stronger our relationship bond becomes.

Why Sex Is Good for the Brain

During sex and orgasm, the brain receives the best chemicals a brain can receive – psychedelic substances that flood it with feelings of pleasure, euphoria, calmness, joy, uplift, vitality, passion, empathy, security, peace, trust, generosity, affection and attachment. So many chemicals, so many sensations, so much health! Sex and intimacy are good for our physical health no less than they are good for the health of a long-term relationship. The wonderful substances that drench the brain during sex and masturbation raise an individual's mood and reduce stress.

When oxytocin is released, the stress hormone cortisol declines. Cortisol is the "silent killer" that causes a lot of damage to our body in times of chronic stress. It acts on all the body systems when we are under pressure and prepares them to cope – to fight, flee or freeze in place. In a state of chronic stress and the body's constant readiness for danger – a danger that usually exists mainly in our heads – the body's systems wear out, the immune system is suppressed and we are more exposed to diseases both from within and without.

The immune system also plays an important role in protecting our brain cells. There are cells of the immune system that perform operations necessary for ongoing maintenance, detoxification and the regeneration and renewal of the neurons in the brain. When we are under stress, the immune system is weakened and the brain does not receive this maintenance and proper damage repair. Every day, brain cells die naturally, and as we age and the immune system weakens, the number of cells that are damaged increases over time and brain function begins to decline. Stress weakens the immune system even more, causing an increase in the erosion processes in the brain and faster ageing. To prevent this situation we must reduce our stress levels. This is why it is important to practise relaxed breathing and/or meditation, to sleep well, eat well and increase oxytocin (through hugs, caresses and orgasms), which also promotes a healthy appetite and good sleep. Sleep after orgasm is generally better.

Brain scans reveal that many different areas of the brain are active during sex. If comparing scans of the areas of the brain that are active during sex with those that are active during sports, we can see that the brain is more intensively active during the former, thanks to the wealth of stimuli received. This state of intense activity is excellent for the brain. It increases the processes of regeneration and damage repair by the immune system and new neurons are created.

Studies have found that with each orgasm, enormous amounts of energy and building materials reach the brain. These include substances such as vitamin A and E, which build neurotransmitters in the brain – aspartic acid, choline, tryptophan and tyrosine – without which the brain cannot grow new neurons, create new connections or, in other words, think. The orgasm actually serves as a kind of massage for the brain, which is soothing yet stimulating, and allows it to work better. In conclusion, here are two important tips for maintaining a long life for the brain into old age: maintain a high frequency of sexual activity throughout your life (either with a partner or solo) and do lots of crosswords and Sudoku. You can vary the activities if you like.

Sex and Prostate Cancer

In a study conducted at the Boston School of Public Health, the frequency of ejaculation, whether through masturbation or intercourse, of 32,000 men was examined and correlated to their chances of contracting prostate cancer, the most common cancer in men over the age of 50 and the third leading cause of death in England. The study concluded that in order to reduce the risk of prostate cancer by a third, men need 21 orgasms a month.

The reason is related to the structure of the male reproductive system. In the seminiferous tube that runs along the penis, at any given moment there are 360 million sperm cells ready to be sent for release. If these hundreds of millions are not sent on their way within three days, they return to the prostate gland, which is responsible for the production of seminal fluid, and there they are absorbed back into the tissues. This process is not favourable for the body and may produce local inflammation and result in damage if this is repeatedly the case over many years. To prevent this kind of damage from occurring in the first place and to encourage sperm to get out into the world so that the body's supply can be replenished, on the fourth day, the man may begin to be troubled by thoughts of sex and wet dreams, with the aim of encouraging him to discharge the old load of sperm through masturbation, or better yet, through sexual intercourse. Every sperm must have his day; that's the motto of the male sexual system, and the reason that men's sex drive is often higher than women's.

Men think about sex on average five times more than women do. Globally, men are also hundreds of per cent more likely to indulge in porn consumption, sex services, sex addiction and sexual harassment. In contrast, women's sex drive is more affected by the monthly increase in oestrogen levels around the time of ovulation and also undergoes changes during pregnancy, childbirth and when raising small children. This is due to the presence of hormones relating to childbirth, breastfeeding and raising children, such as the hormone prolactin, which causes a decrease in sex drive and increases the tendency to nurture. Moreover, since women experience two to three times more stress and anxiety than men, they also report a greater decrease in sex drive due to the suppressive effect of cortisol.

The Legendary Female Orgasm

The common assumption regarding the purpose of the female orgasm is that it contributes to relaxation, reduces pain and stress, and assists conception. The mucus secreted during orgasm lines the cervix and speeds the sperm on their way toward the uterus. Regarding the exact amount of orgasms needed for women's health, there are still no exact numbers, but research shows that women who are sexually active near menopause suffer less from menopause symptoms than women who are not. Studies on the use of sex toys among women show positive changes in blood flow, muscle tone in the vaginal tissues, improved sexual arousal, sexual desire and satisfaction, increased orgasmic pleasure and reduced sexual distress.

The female orgasm has enjoyed a semi-mythical status since ancient times. According to Greek legend, Tiresias was a priest of Zeus, who was punished by Hera, Zeus's consort, and sentenced to live seven years as a woman. One day after this, Tiresias joined in a heated argument between Zeus and Hera over who enjoys sex more – the man or the woman? Hera claimed that the man had more fun and Zeus argued for the woman. Since Tiresias had experienced both sides, he averred that the woman enjoys sex nine times more than the man. For this answer, Hera struck him blind.

Tiresias was partly right: women don't have one single type of orgasm like men do. Women experience two types of orgasms. One originates from the external stimulation of the upper part of the clitoris, while the second type of orgasm is caused by penetration into the vagina. In both types of stimulation, different blood flow can be measured and it seems that this variance creates the difference in sensation between the two kinds.

There are weaker orgasms and there are stronger orgasms, but what contributes to the strength of the female orgasm? In 2009, Dr Stephanie Ortig, a neuropsychologist from Syracuse University in New York, tested the difference between the quality of orgasms of women who were in love with their partner against the quality of orgasms of women who were not. To test first whether the women were truly in love, Ortig tracked their brainwaves upon hearing their partner's name mentioned. Women in love display different brain activity to women who are not in love; in women in love, the area of the emotional brain called the insula, a part associated with obsessive behaviour and addiction, is more active.

In the second step, Ortig analysed their reports of orgasms and their intensity, and saw, not surprisingly, that the more in love the woman was, the more she experienced powerful orgasms. There is a correlation between love and quality orgasms, of course, thanks to oxytocin, the love hormone, which increases the intensity of an orgasm. In addition, Ortig discovered that in the women in love, there was increased activity during orgasm in the area of the brain that relates to creating and retrieving memories, which intensifies the pleasure. Basically, the women in love experienced a strong orgasm, stored it as a pleasant memory and then recalled it the next time they were with their partner. The oxytocin released in the orgasm creates the bonding, which gets stronger with each orgasm.

Another study that examined the relationship between the quality of female orgasms and the degree of attraction to a partner found that partners of men whose faces are more symmetrical report more powerful orgasms. Symmetry, as mentioned earlier, is an indication of genetic qualities, and it seems that the orgasm also favours a genetic quality.

Female versus Male Orgasms

When considering the anatomy of the male sexual system, the ease with which a man experiences orgasm and the similarity in orgasms between different men, it appears that the system is almost the same in every man. While there are differences between different men, these are negligible and do not approach the complexity of the female reproductive system and the variation in orgasm from woman to woman. For women, orgasm is a multi-layered and idiosyncratic affair. The difference and complexity in women may be due to the fact that it is men, not women, who are under enormous evolutionary pressure to spread their sperm – as much sperm, as quickly as possible – since they cannot bring offspring into the world by themselves and they are never sure which offspring are really theirs. In such a situation, simplicity, efficiency and speed must come at the expense of variety and complexity.

In contrast, since women are the ones who bear the entire burden of pregnancy and care from a biological point of view, it is evolutionarily important that they develop clever and complex mechanisms to make sure that their genes mix with the best genes available. If you are a heterosexual woman looking for a partner with whom to raise children, you should take your time over making your choice because once his sperm has met your egg, there will be no going back. In this sense, a multidimensional and sometimes stealthy orgasm is an excellent mechanism.

Women tend to fall more deeply in love with men who pleasure them into orgasm. The amount of oxytocin released by a woman during orgasm is responsible for this. Oestrogen, the female sex hormone, increases the secretion of oxytocin and therefore the level of oxytocin in the blood of a woman is usually two to three times higher than the level of oxytocin in the blood of a man at any given time. In addition, testosterone, which is found at much higher concentrations in men's blood than in women's, has been found to inhibit the action of oxytocin and, as early as puberty, inhibits the communication and empathy centres in a boy's brain compared to that of a girl. Researchers in Japan have even proved that testosterone inhibits the action of oxytocin and suppresses parental behaviour in male mice.

Is it the higher level of oxytocin in the blood of women with oestrogen, compared to the lower level of oxytocin in the blood of men due to testosterone, that causes women to bond after sex more than men? Is this why men are more likely to seek thrills? If we look at the brain, it seems that there are differences in the areas activated and the substances secreted in a man's brain compared to a woman's brain during intercourse. Areas relating to the physical sensation of sexual contact and to processing visual images, and the amygdala, which is linked to the management of emotions, are very active in the male brain. The levels of aggression and sexual stimulation that arise under the influence of testosterone are greater in men, while in a woman's brain, there is a decrease in activity in areas related to anxiety and stress, and an awakening of the amygdala and other emotional areas. The frontal lobe, the area of judgement, turns off in men shortly after the sexual stimulation of the brain, and in women almost only at the moment of orgasm. Furthermore, the flow of oxytocin in orgasm is higher in the woman, while the man receives a higher dose of dopamine.

Understanding what happens to our brains during sex can explain a great deal of the behavioural differences we observe in women and men. Due to the high levels of dopamine and adrenaline that are released in a man's brain from the effect of testosterone on the amygdala, men are more addicted than women to sex and porn. A higher dopamine level is obtained when the signal is new – that is, someone new – and therefore men are more inclined than women to have multiple partners. Also, the inflammation of the larger amygdala in men is related to the fact that men are more stimulated than women by violent acts.

From the perspective of the brain, the same gland, the amygdala, is involved in sexual stimulation and aggression; therefore violence and sex are linked in the animal kingdom. Sex in the animal kingdom is usually not performed to the sounds of gentle violins but is a violent act in which the male subdues the female and fights other males in the process. In some species, if the act is not violent, ovulation does not occur. In geese, for example, only a decent bite from the gander on the goose's neck when he mounts her will cause the egg to leave the goose's ovary and head for the uterus. There is no fertilization without violence.

In addition to these differences, in the male orgasm, higher levels of vasopressin are released compared to the oxytocin released during the female orgasm. As mentioned, vasopressin is the male version of oxytocin, which encourages more territorial behaviour, marking out and aggressively defending the territory against other males. This is in stark contrast to the desire for attachment and nurturing behaviour that oxytocin encourages. Moreover, testosterone also plays a role in the creation of territorial aggression in males. Researchers at the University of Massachusetts have shown how testosterone regulates vasopressin receptors in the male brain and increases territorial behaviour linked to the hormone. In humans, too, men are more prone to territoriality and jealousy where a woman is concerned, sometimes obsessively so.

Many men report that they are turned on sexually by a woman's admiration of their physical abilities and their penis. This phenomenon of sexual arousal following admiration is not unique to humans and is known in some quarters as the "cichlid effect", after the fish in which the phenomenon was also observed. Male cichlid fish become sexually aroused only if a female, who enters their territory and watches them, shows a gesture of appreciation. The female lays her eggs near the male who manages to impress her thanks to his size, his appearance and his aggressive behaviour toward any other males who stray into his territory.

A Question of Nature or Nurture

So, are the various stereotypes about men and women real and based on hormonal differences, neurons and the interests of the male and female genes? Or are we humans not at all similar to rats and mice but a product of our environment, education and culture? There is no single answer to this.

As far as the emotional (limbic) brain is concerned, more remains unknown about it than has been revealed. Significant developments in brain research have only become possible in recent decades, thanks to technological breakthroughs such as MRI brain scanners, the ability to read brainwaves with EEG technology and the latest advance in this field called optogenetics – a combination of physics, genetics and brain research. It is a precise method of stimulating the brains of animals for research through genetic engineering and the use of optical fibres. Optogenetics makes it possible to turn on or off a single neuron or a network of neurons in the brain, and see how the organism reacts and changes its behaviour in real time. Before 2012, neuroscientists couldn't have dreamed of looking into the brain in real time and seeing which neurons activate which behaviour or function.

It is important to note, however, that of the various brain structures, the emotional-limbic brain has not been the subject of extensive study, mainly because most of the significant research is carried out on animals, and until a few decades ago the prevailing assumption in science was that animals do not have emotions – that emotions are unique to humans and set us apart from the rest of the animal kingdom. When it became apparent that other mammals have emotions that are fundamentally similar to the ones we experience, emotions mediated by the same chemicals and producing similar behaviours – joy, sadness, love, hate, friendliness, depression, anxiety, stress – researchers began to study the emotions and behaviour of these animals, too. From these studies, we can glean quite a lot about the biology of animal behaviour, which is basically similar to ours. The difference with humans lies in our control and regulation of emotions and behaviour, which are done by the new frontal lobe.

Another new and ground-breaking field, which is related to brain research and is constantly growing, is the field of neuro-epigenetics. This is a fascinating area that examines the effect of stimuli and factors from the environment on the expression of genes inside nerve cells; in other words, how stimuli from the environment affect the neurons and the creation of wiring in the brain and the nervous system in general. Significant epigenetic changes occur during foetal development following stimuli in the womb, as well as at the beginning of life through stimuli from an infant's parents and their surroundings. There is now evidence that some epigenetic changes can be passed from generation to generation through different pathways of paternal and maternal epigenetic inheritance. These new findings are fascinating and are changing everything we know about heredity and evolution.

There is no doubt that as a result of these accelerated developments in brain research and genetics, in the coming decades we will reach a much deeper understanding of the biology of emotions and the effect of neurochemicals, hormones and genes on the variety of emotions, and consequently also on human behaviour with its many characteristics.

Falling Hard – The Side Effects of Love

At the beginning of a relationship, a couple's orgasms are on fire. The brain experiences new and intoxicating stimuli from a new partner. The entire nervous system is in ecstasy, and the brain is flooded with all the delightful psychedelic love drugs we've considered. However, as we all know, drugs can have serious side effects, so what, if any, are the side effects of love, what causes them and when do they pass?

Let's start with the side effects caused by the strongest drug of all, dopamine, the pleasure hormone. When we fall in love, the brain is drenched in dopamine. Every look, touch, caress and, of course, sexual encounter and orgasm releases huge amounts of dopamine; the brain is getting high. The sensations are of supreme pleasure, powerful euphoria, bursts of energy and arousal. In order for us to remember what makes us feel good and then act to receive it, dopamine greatly increases the activity in the memory areas, so that the pleasure is seared into everything that reminds us of it. Conditioning is created between the sight, smell, touch, voice and messages of the loved one and that pleasure, and a process of addiction begins. We find ourselves strongly motivated to relive this pleasure.

Falling in love is fundamentally a certain type of addiction, be that an addiction to the object of our desire or to the very essence of love itself, to the feeling of loving and being loved. When you are together you feel on top of the world, with feelings of euphoria and pleasure, but when you are not together withdrawal symptoms appear: depression, nervousness, anxiety, fatigue, lack of sleep, lack of appetite, disturbing thoughts, lack of concentration, decreased attention and decreased energy. The depth of the "down" matches the peak of the "high". Depression, sadness and anxiety are also caused by a decrease in serotonin, the happy hormone, which occurs when we are removed from the object of our love. We find ourselves on a roller coaster of positive and negative emotions.

If we are unlucky, these disturbing thoughts can attain the status of OCD, obsessive-compulsive disorder. In this instance, the condition is clinically known as "relationship OCD" (ROCD), an obsessive-compulsive disorder specifically concerned with relationships, which causes damage to the daily functioning of the person in love. The disorder is characterized by an obsessive preoccupation with the object of affection and the relationship with them. Annoying thoughts like "Does he want/love me?" and "Why didn't she call or text?" raise doubts about the relationship: *Does he, doesn't he? Is this it, or not?* There may be an obsessive preoccupation with the loved one's perceived qualities and frequent consultation with family members and friends regarding the relationship, to the point of compulsive behaviour. Following the partner, snooping through his/her phone and emails, trying to check who else he/she's been seen with, and what they're wearing . . . This disorder causes a lot of stress and anxiety, which may cause damage to the relationship as well as to future relationships. In these cases, it is important for the individual to receive guidance and treatment so as not to sabotage their relationships generally.

Another phenomenon that characterizes the mind in love is viewing relationships through rose-tinted glasses. When we are falling in love, everything appears rosy to us because of oxytocin. The love hormone causes us to see our partner as simply perfect at first, our soulmate, the one we've been waiting for all our lives. Oxytocin makes us focus on their positive qualities and remove any negative values from our field of vision. When these initial hormones and chemicals subside and the magic wears off, the partner's negative qualities suddenly emerge and we ask ourselves why we didn't see them as they really are earlier on, because it was right in front of our eyes the whole time. They say that love is blind, and that is certainly the motto of oxytocin: how on Earth would we fall in love if we could see reality exactly as it is? And if that's not enough, serotonin joins in, and both hormones cause us to have illusions about our partner and the relationship.

Jealousy, the Green-Eyed Monster

Jealousy is another powerful side effect of falling in love. It is said that jealousy is blind, perhaps because it too is the result of the same love hormone, oxytocin, distorting our vision. In the ancient Hebrew paean to love, the Song of Songs, we read, "Fierce as death is love, as hard as jealousy." We are definitely dealing with a tough hormone. In the context of romantic relationships, jealousy is actually a form of anxiety that the partner will fall in love with someone else. It can be experienced as pain, a knife that slices through the body, if we see our partner being loving toward or, heaven forbid, having sexual contact with someone else.

The jealousy mechanism has an evolutionary logic, or it would not have remained with us. It serves to preserve a long-term relationship that is fundamentally based on a meeting between two unrelated strangers, with fully developed minds, who are trying to create a strong bond that entails self-sacrifice and commitment in the hope that this will last a lifetime. This bond involves oxytocin and the other chemicals of love and it therefore makes sense to prevent your partner from producing the same hormones and chemicals with someone else: after all, if our lover were to produce the love hormones in connection with someone else on a regular basis, he or she might fall in love with that person and leave us, and what then would happen to our offspring? (And even if there are no offspring, what then would become of us?)

However, like all other emotions and the chemicals that produce them, jealousy does not come from a rational part of the brain but from the irrational part, so it can also reach levels of madness. A certain amount of jealousy can be used to spice up a relationship – the feeling that our partner is jealous of us can give us the sense that we are wanted and desired, which is an empowering message for our ego to receive. But if the jealousy becomes obsessive, one partner in the relationship may eventually feel suffocated, insecure and forced to repeatedly prove his or her loyalty, love and devotion, as if trapped in an endless test. In such a situation, jealousy may become a self-fulfilling prophecy and the anxiety of abandonment will become a reality, not because the partner has fallen in love with someone else but because of the stress and feelings of distress.

Obsessive jealousy stems from a need for control, not from love for one's partner. It is an expression of a desire for control over a partner, and also a fear of dependence. The area of the brain that is responsible for regulating feelings of jealousy is, of course, the frontal lobe. But the more hardships, disappointments and stress we have experienced in our previous relationships, as well as in our dealings with our family in our early years, the more difficult it will be for our frontal lobe to regulate the destructive feelings of jealousy and anxiety that can arise when we fall in love. Since it is difficult for our emotional brain to free itself from strong conditioning created around feelings of distress linked to love, it may be necessary for us to seek professional support to stop obsessive jealousy not only jeopardizing our relationship, but our mental and physical health, too.

The Tragedy of Love

A story that demonstrates the power of the love drugs and their side effects involves a dolphin and a woman. Sometime in the 1960s, NASA scientists decided to teach dolphins to understand English and thus communicate with humans. To test this bright idea, they built a large aquarium in the US Virgin Islands and placed in it a young dolphin named Peter and his custodian, 23-year-old Margaret Lovatt.

Peter and Margaret lived at the pool for three months. In the mornings she taught him English and at night she slept on a bunk by the pool so he could see her. Two weeks later, English was the last thing on Peter's mind. He had fallen head over heels in love with Margaret. He just wanted to be with her, to hear her, to play with her. Dolphins are very sociable mammals who normally live in a school. But when Peter was brought dolphin friends to play with, an activity he usually liked very much, he was hostile toward them. He became jealous and violent, wouldn't let Margaret get close to another dolphin, wouldn't let any other dolphin get close to her and wouldn't rest until they were removed.

Peter was flooded with love drugs, head over heels in love. If he had been asked and he really could have answered, he likely would have said he wanted to live with Margaret for ever. He was sexually aroused most of the time, under the influence of oxytocin, and wanted to rub against her constantly, unable to concentrate on anything else. After a while, the NASA scientists realized that the experiment was not progressing in the desired direction, since Peter had only learned to respond to a few words of English. At the end of the first month, the project was stopped and the two were separated. Peter was transferred to another aquarium and Margaret left to continue her life.

Poor Peter experienced a deep heartbreak and displayed all the withdrawal symptoms that follow the cessation of the supply of love drugs. He sank into a deep depression, became apathetic, stopped eating and after two weeks committed suicide; he dived and never resurfaced. Peter's tragic story demonstrates the power of love drugs and the preservation of the age-old oxytocin mechanism and the emotional-limbic brain among the various mammals. Needless to say, NASA received sharp criticism for the experiment and animal rights organizations filed lawsuits against the organization for animal abuse.

Humans as well as dolphins commit suicide in the name of love. There is a saying that falling in love is like pointing a gun at your head; the power of love should never be underestimated. According to the Centers for Disease Control and Prevention (CDC) in the US, relationship problems are the leading cause of suicide, accounting for more than 40 per cent of deaths. This chilling finding is perhaps the most dramatic illustration yet of the powerful impact relationships can have on our physical, emotional and spiritual well-being. It is easy to conjecture the evolutionary reason that humans pay so much attention to relationships; we are, after all, very social animals. It is also easy to understand why even the threat of being alone is enough to create such great stress that it would cause a person to take their own life. The truth is that we humans become sick with loneliness and healthy with love.

Broken Heart Syndrome

Due to the fact that we are creatures who crave connection, separation from a partner is experienced by our nervous system as a high-level threat to our survival, and this activates the stress response in full force. The amygdala – the stress- and emotion-management gland – sends messengers to the adrenal gland and orders it to release cortisol and adrenaline into the bloodstream, which affects every cell in the body and prepares it to fight.

The adrenaline that floods the blood circulation causes the heart rate to accelerate; the small blood vessels of the heart contract, which leads to a temporary lack of blood supply to the heart. In response, the "cerebellum" of the heart or the cardiac nervous system, which consists of 40,000 neurons, sends messages of pain and distress to the brain, which is why we feel heartache. This condition can cause physical damage to the heart tissue and the death of heart muscle cells, which can lead to scarring of the heart and irreversible damage. The term for this phenomenon is "takotsubo cardiomyopathy", first described in Japan in 1990. Takotsubo are Japanese octopus traps resembling the shape of a damaged heart.

In response to the intensity of the stress of separation, the survival reactions are activated – fight, flight, freeze or an attempt to "tend and befriend":

The fight strategy can be expressed by attacking the partner, venting anger, and threatening and unleashing aggression. "Fight" can also be expressed by being aggressive to anyone else who happens to be around, including friends and family. Unfortunately, part of our automatic calming mechanism during times of stress is to take out our aggression on someone else, and we find it relaxing. Stress also suppresses empathy; when we feel bad we don't see the other and don't care who we are hurting in that moment. Later come the guilty feelings, which increase the stress.

The flight strategy often manifests itself in escaping into other pursuits, such as working from morning until night, intense physical activity, quickly going on dates and meeting someone new, surrounding ourselves with friends, partying or experimenting with addictive substances to cloud the mind and ease the chronic mental pain.

The freeze strategy can appear as helplessness, falling into depression, a reluctance to get out of bed, the loss of desire and the motivation to move. A freeze situation can sometimes result in a person getting stuck in the same situation for a long time, with no desire to meet new people, so as not to get hurt again.

The strategy of "tend and befriend", sometimes referred to as "fawning", sees a person trying to please and appease their partner, making promises and returning to them again and again.

Most of us will practise a combination of these strategies during a breakup. However, in people who are particularly sensitive to stress, characteristics of OCD such as obsessive disturbing thoughts and compulsive behaviour can also occur following separation.

Why can our reaction to a breakup be so strong? A relationship split can be experienced as such an acute pain because it instantly denies us the calming action of the love hormone, oxytocin, on the vagus nerve. The end of the relationship takes away from us the hugs, touch, kisses, laughter, conversation, the supporting shoulder, the protection and the partnership that combine to calm our nervous system. Instead, we may find ourselves in a state of loneliness, which can cause stress. According to Professor Julianne Holt-Lunstad from Utah, loneliness can do as much damage to our body as smoking 15 cigarettes a day.

How Do You Heal a Broken Heart?

As Rabbi Kfir Shahar once said: "Love is the only medicine in the world whose side effects are much more serious than the disease it is supposed to solve." So how do you heal from heartbreak? One of the most important things during a breakup is to create as many support systems as possible and use the healing power of empathic friends on the vagus nerve to get ourselves out of survival mode. When we share with other people what we are going through and describe our feelings, the frontal lobe of the brain works together with the emotional brain, and the event is processed and transferred from the short-term memory (the amygdala) to the long-term memory. After we have given voice to our thoughts, we immediately feel more in control and calmer. In this context, crying is very healing because it allows us to release trapped negative emotions linked to the event that we may otherwise try to repress on a daily basis. Crying allows for maximum processing and release, after which we feel much calmer.

Women often have more support systems in place than men do; they tend to share more of their feelings with others. Because men are less likely to talk about what they are going through and thereby process their negative experiences, they can suffer more from latent or hidden depression. Women, on the other hand, are more prone to excessive preoccupation with negative thoughts, or overthinking. This is called a tendency to rumination, or repetitive negative thinking. This is one of the main reasons that women suffer two to three times more than men do from depression and anxiety.

To help prevent this, here are some important tips to help us say goodbye to relationships that don't work out:

- Don't fight your negative emotions. You will be flooded with difficult feelings – of sadness, sorrow, grief and anger. Give them space, because suppressing and ignoring them will only prolong the time it takes for you to heal and may even cause more emotional blockages and avoidance.
- Talk openly with people about your feelings. Accept the inevitable fact that breakups are an integral part of any love life. Try as much as possible to limit any thoughts of regret, guilt or self-flagellation, as these destructive feelings will only cause you to wallow in self-pity.
- Connect to your pillars of happiness – whatever makes you feel good, such as music, dance, sports, travel, sun, sea, friends, family and pets.

- As far as possible, create a new healthy lifestyle without your ex. Avoid falling into negative patterns of thinking. In an attempt to protect itself, the mind creates thought patterns to try to avoid pain, such as "all men (or all women) are the same", "you can't trust anyone", and "there's no love out there, only self-interest". However, these patterns have a tendency to reinforce themselves and become limiting beliefs that can make our future relationships more difficult.
- There is no failure – there is only growth and learning. Focus on what you learned about yourself from your last dating experience.
- Sometimes it's hard to do this alone. If you feel you are stuck in negative thought patterns, get help from professionals. We all need help.

It's important to remember that the scars on the heart do not simply disappear; we carry them with us all our lives as badges of honour. Every time we meet a potential new partner and forge a fresh relationship, we bring into that relationship a bundle of painful scars caused by our past experiences. As we know, the brain remembers negative events at least three times more vividly than positive ones, which means that certain traits or behaviours associated with our previous partners will get burned into our brain, along with any triggers connected to them.

From an evolutionary point of view, this is a survival learning mechanism designed to prevent sentient beings from repeating past mistakes. But today this mechanism can make us unnecessarily careful, avoidant, afraid and defensive. There is a need for conscious work, a corrective transformation, to disconnect ourselves from our conditioning, so that we do not remain prisoners of our past, repeating the same negative experiences and becoming trapped in a state of exhaustion.

Types of Attachment

The imprinting process – that fast and powerful learning at the beginning of life, when the qualities of caring parents are seared into our minds to enable attachment – affects not only the way we choose partners later on, but also how we bond with them, and what form that attachment will take. Attachment, as defined by the psychiatrist John Bowlby, is a baby's innate inclination to seek the proximity of its parents and to feel protected and safe in their presence. This is based on an evolutionary survival need and remains a fundamental part of a person's mental makeup throughout that individual's life.

Different attachment styles are formed during the first year of infancy and tend to remain consistent throughout a person's life.

A safe attachment style develops in those people who received a consistent response to their needs in infancy, which created a relationship model based on the belief and trust that the caregiver would always be there for them.

In contrast, an anxious attachment style develops when an infant receives an inconsistent response to his or her needs, which creates anxiety and greater dependency on the figure of the caregiver. Those with this attachment style feel insecure and distrustful of relationships. It is difficult for them to support others because they are busy looking for support for themselves. They create dependent relationships, fear that they are not loved, generate quite a few relationship dramas and generally feel more anxiety, depression and anger.

An avoidant attachment style develops in those individuals whose needs were not met at all in infancy. They learned to become self-reliant and not to trust people. Those with an avoidant attachment style tend to be suspicious and don't like to feel dependent on their partner. They keep a safe distance and don't always correctly assess when their partner needs them. They have difficulty coping with their partner's expectations and shy away from intimacy, for fear that could lead to their partner exerting control over them. They do not betray their anxiety and anger; rather, they avoid revealing their feelings.

Ironically, those with an anxious attachment style tend to be attracted to those with an avoidant attachment style and vice versa. So when the two dance together, it's an unhappy match in which one is never able to satisfy the other's needs and it usually ends in tears.

Is it possible to change our attachment style? Due to the way our brains are shaped at the beginning of life, the answer is no, but through awareness and therapy, we can learn to adapt behaviours from the safe attachment style and repair aspects of insecure attachment styles formed in our very earliest relationships. This approach can help build a person's sense of identity, strength and autonomy, which will ultimately help them to find a partner and enjoy their own happy ending.

CHAPTER 5

WHEN TWO BECOMES THREE

According to statistics, for most married couples the crises commence around three years after the arrival of the first child. Taking care of the children and the transition to a family configuration completely changes marital harmony. The changes are not only psychological but also biological. Let's examine how the biology within the family affects the relationship.

A man is walking in a meadow and sees two horses munching grass in front of him. How does he know if they are related? If the man offers hay to the horses and one horse moves the hay toward the other's mouth and lets it eat first, he will immediately know that this is a mother and her foal. This ancient Chinese parable sums up the essence of motherhood. But what drives a mother to place the needs of her offspring before her own?

All creatures are born selfish, programmed to take care of their own needs first. However, as soon as she becomes a mother, massive changes in her nervous system cause a female to prioritize the needs of her offspring – a form of reprogramming, if you like, the purpose of which is to ensure the survival of her young and the safe transfer of genes to the next generation. Since 97 per cent of animal mothers on Earth are single parents, virtually all animal life on this planet depends on a mother's attachment, devotion and care for her offspring.

An instructive example is found in the giant Pacific octopus. In most species of octopus, the female digests the male's neurons while mating with him. Afterwards, he collapses and dies. However, in species such as the giant Pacific octopus, the males have developed tactics to avoid the predatory females, and when the female approaches, he pretty much throws his sperm packet at her and scarpers. The female octopus looks for an empty cave in which to lay her billion eggs and for six whole months will not move from the cave, guarding the eggs, moving her tentacles from side to side, supplying them with oxygen and cleaning them from accumulations of harmful fungi. For half a year, she does not go out to look for food and eventually she dies of hunger. With her last ounce of strength, she blows water over the eggs to hasten their hatching. They come out into the world, feed on the decaying remains of their dead mother, and set off into the great wide yonder. Out of the billion eggs, only a few will make it to maturity and they owe their lives to the mother octopus.

Similar dramatic changes in the behaviour of females after pregnancy and birth can be seen throughout the animal kingdom. These changes originate from the processes that occur in the female's brain during pregnancy and birth, changes at a tissue level, neuron level and at a gene level through epigenetics (changes in gene expression resulting from external or environmental factors). It is a fascinating example of neuroplasticity – the incredible flexibility of the brain.

The centre of the mother's brain goes through some very dramatic reorganization and structural changes during pregnancy, with changes in the grey matter containing the nuclei of the neurons whose role is to process sensory or movement stimuli. These changes occur in areas that are involved in understanding social interactions, creating attachment and which are responsible for the ability to empathize.

Studies have shown these changes improve the mother's ability to understand the baby's nonverbal communications through facial expressions and types of crying, which in turn helps the baby understand the world around it, and how to regulate its internal stimuli. Animal studies demonstrate how changes in brain wiring during pregnancy provide essential adaptations within the mother, which increase her mental and emotional focus on the helpless creature that enters her life.

A mother's brain changes significantly and to a large extent also irreversibly. Researchers from Leiden University in the Netherlands recorded with scans (fMRI) the changes in the brains of mothers: during pregnancy, before the birth, immediately after it and two years later. They saw significant and long-term changes in the brain, so much so that a computer program was able to predict with 100 per cent accuracy, based on a brain scan image, whether a woman had experienced pregnancy in the past. Attachment tests were also used to examine the emotional and social patterns of the baby and the mother, and the researchers found that the higher the level of structural changes in the mother's brain, the higher the level of attachment to her baby.

One of the most fascinating studies in my opinion, which provides a rare glimpse into a mother's mind and demonstrates the differences between male and female brains, was carried out on mice by Professor Tali Kimchi and her research team from the Weizmann Institute of Science in Israel. During pregnancy, a mouse – also a single parent – begins to build a nest with sawdust and cotton wool in preparation for her offspring. (This nesting behaviour also occurs in pregnant women, preparing the house for the upcoming birth, and is a product of hormonal changes involving oestrogen, progesterone and prolactin.) After her litter is born, the mouse keeps the pups close to her in the nest, bringing them back to it when they move away and licking them intensely. This is maternal behaviour.

The researchers then took some newborn pups and transferred them to an empty cage, where they installed a partial partition and arranged a nest of cotton wool and sawdust across the partition. The researchers put a foreign mouse, which was also a mother having delivered a litter of her own a few hours earlier, into the empty half of the cage. The "stepmother" immediately collected the pups, one after the other, crossed the partition and placed them in the cotton wool nest, where she guarded them and licked them. In short, this mouse displayed maternal behaviour. In the next step, the researchers placed newborn pups in a cage with a virgin mouse, which had never given birth. After a few hours, she too collected the pups, bypassed the partition, put them in the nest and licked them, displaying the same maternal behaviour. But when the researchers put a male into the cage with the pups, at best he showed indifference toward them and at worst he attacked and killed them.

To understand the cause of the different behaviour, the researchers examined the brains of the mice, where they found changes in areas associated with pleasure. They noticed that the pleasure system in the brain of the virgin female had a higher number of neurons that are responsible for the secretion of the hormone oxytocin (the love hormone) than the brain of the male. However, the most significant change was observed in the mother's brain, where the number of oxytocin-secreting neurons doubled at the time of giving birth to her own pups and was therefore double the number of those in the brain of the virgin mouse. That is, during childbirth, the number of neurons which are responsible for the secretion of oxytocin is doubled in the pleasure system of the mother's brain. This change is irreversible and actually leads to increased pleasure and thus motivation for showing nurturing behaviour toward the pups.

The Mother of Hormones

Oxytocin is the hormone that creates motherhood; it orchestrates the creation of life, nourishment and nurturing. The highest levels of oxytocin are found in the blood of a female giving birth. It promotes childbirth by causing the contraction of the uterine muscles and it governs breastfeeding through the contraction of the mammary glands. This hormone has remained surprisingly conserved throughout evolution.

At the very start of pregnancy, oxytocin is secreted from the woman's pituitary gland into her bloodstream, causing changes in her metabolism, with the aim of storing energy in her body in the form of fat, to satisfy the demands of the developing foetus. During the third trimester of pregnancy, the oxytocin levels in the mother's blood will already be significantly higher than before, and will affect her behaviour. The expectant mother will become more open and sociable toward friends and acquaintances and will strengthen ties with parents and other family members.

At the end of the ninth month, the moment arrives when she will not be able to provide the foetus in her womb with more than 20 per cent of the nourishment it needs. The birth process actually begins with the baby's own hunger pangs. The hunger felt by the foetus stimulates its own pituitary gland to secrete increasing doses of oxytocin which, through their shared circulation, will reach the mother's brain. In response, the mother will also secrete larger doses of oxytocin, causing contractions of the uterine muscles, and thus the labour begins. (Pitocin, the induction hormone that is sometimes administered to induce labour, is actually synthetic oxytocin that helps the uterus contract.) Even after the birth, at any time of distress, the baby will release oxytocin when crying so that the mother, or any other person, will come to meet the infant's needs.

The rush of oxytocin that floods the mother's body during childbirth also goes some way toward easing the pain, as it causes the release of endorphins which help to numb sensations of pain.

Immediately after birth, exhausted and hungry, the baby will be placed on the mother's stomach where he will instinctively grope for her nipples. The contact with the nipple sends nerve messages to the mother's brain to secrete more oxytocin, which shrinks the mammary glands and allows milk to flow into the baby's mouth. In these moments of breastfeeding, oxytocin will evoke strong feelings of closeness and euphoria. The skin-to-skin contact causes an increased secretion of oxytocin in both baby and mother and their bond begins to tighten.

Oxytocin also causes increased activity in the long-term memory areas (the hippocampus) so that in these moments the smell, touch, taste, voice and other features belonging to each other become engraved in the brains of both the baby and its mother. This begins a few moments after birth and continues for the first few days, and is part of the imprinting process, creating an unbreakable bond between the offspring and its mother so that it can recognize her and seek her closeness, protection and nourishment. The bond also creates a sense of obligation in the mother toward her offspring. The connection between them will grow stronger with every glance, hug, caress, kiss, smile, laugh, kind word, compliment and moment of empathy.

However, along with feelings of closeness and euphoria, the mother may well also experience moments of depression and sadness. The sharp drop in oestrogen and progesterone levels after childbirth can cause her to experience mood changes, while the stress hormone cortisol that is also secreted can produce anxiety and depression. The mother's lack of sleep will further contribute to her increased levels of stress and depression. More than half of new mothers experience various types of depression after giving birth. One in seven women will experience a state of clinical depression, also known as postpartum depression.

Childbirth is traumatic for both mind and body. When the woman's experience is overwhelming and her mind is flooded with stimuli that she has difficulty containing and processing, this overload can cause a disruption in the secretion of oxytocin. This disruption in turn may cause the mother to shut down and withdraw into herself, avoiding stimuli that remind her of the trauma. Postpartum depression can manifest itself as sadness, lack of energy, helplessness, exhaustion, a feeling of emptiness, outbursts of anger, difficulty caring for the baby (from showing little interest in her offspring to excessive concern), sleep disorders, eating disorders and a sharp decrease in libido. Situations of extreme overprotection or disinterest in the baby may also cause a disruption in the attachment process.

Postpartum depression is a very common phenomenon, but half of the cases are not diagnosed at all and go untreated in many women. Interestingly, the condition is more common in the industrialized West than in traditional tribal societies. This is because in the individualistic Western society, there is often much less support from the extended family and the community than in traditional societies. Many Western women are left alone with their baby for most of the day, which increases their sense of alienation and depression. They may feel that they cannot live up to society's expectation that they should feel intense happiness and be on top of the world, while in reality, they feel exhausted, stressed and lonely. In the West, mothers of toddlers and young children are a high-risk group for clinical depression.

Evolutionarily speaking, we are built to raise offspring in a group like our monkey cousins and other mammals do. An infant chimpanzee, for example, is cared for by an average of four adults, including the mother, as is the case in human tribal societies. In tribal societies, young mothers are almost never left alone. They receive a lot of mental and emotional support from their extended family members, community and more experienced mothers.

What's Happening to Dad?

The hormonal and structural changes that take place in the body and brain of the mother during pregnancy and childbirth do not occur in the body and brain of the father. Many new fathers feel confused and don't know how to deal with the dramatic changes in their lives, nor what is happening to their partners. So how do fathers create their paternal identity, what role does biology play in fatherhood, and how does it affect relationships?

As mentioned, Professor Tali Kimchi's research found that the number of neurons secreting oxytocin in the pleasure system of the brains of male mice was found to be lower when compared to the number in the brain of the virgin female. The behaviour of the male and female was also different, with the virgin female eventually displaying nurturing behaviour, while the male was indifferent to the pups or attacked them. The difference is due to the presence of testosterone, the male hormone. During brain development, testosterone causes a delay in the production of oxytocin and a subsequent delay in the development of the empathy centres in the male's brain.

However, when the researchers injected synthetic oxytocin into the male's brain, his behaviour changed: he picked up the cubs, one by one, bypassed the partition, put them in the nest, guarded them and licked them. The addition of oxytocin altered his behaviour completely.

Most male mammals in the wild do not show parental behaviour toward their offspring and do not bond with them. Testosterone drives males in nature to fight for status, take risks and search for females. Those males who do form a strong and stable bond with their partner and offspring, showing unusual devotion toward them, are the males of rare monogamous species such the prairie voles, which, as we have seen, have undergone genetic changes relating to the love hormones.

So what happened in male humans? Unlike most other mammals, men can form a deep and strong bond with their children and take care of them. How did this fatherly love develop? This is a fascinating and important biological question.

Professor Ruth Feldman from Bar-Ilan University in Israel followed a number of young heterosexual couples for six months after the birth of their first child. She visited their home once a week and measured the increase in oxytocin levels in the blood and saliva of the fathers and the mothers while they were individually caring for the baby. Professor Feldman and her team wanted to know if there was a difference between the increase in the oxytocin level in the father's blood compared to the increase in the mother's blood, during their respective parenting periods. It transpired that although the level of oxytocin in the women's blood was higher, when offering parental care a father's oxytocin level jumped to equal that of the mother, suggesting that fathers bond at a hormonal level with their children through caring for them, playing with them and spending time together.

The researchers noticed another interesting phenomenon, concerning the triangular relationship between the mother, father and baby. When the mother's level of oxytocin is high, so is the father's, but when the mother's level is low, so is the father's. There is a relationship between the caregivers in which the primary caregiver, the one who spends more time with the baby (and in most cases this is the mother), influences the secondary caregiver. The mechanism responsible for this is our old friend the mirror neuron mechanism. The mother and the father are bound together in an emotional connection through their neurons, forming a connection that also affects the baby's brain.

A family is a fascinating and complex neuronal constellation. This is why when women experience postpartum depression, it affects the men who go through it with them. Feldman's study and others like it show that fathers who are emotionally involved in the care of their children also undergo hormonal changes: there is an increase in oxytocin, vasopressin (the male version of oxytocin, which is linked to protection and territoriality) and the hormone prolactin (which encourages nurturing behaviour), a lessening of the sex drive and lower testosterone. These hormonal changes in the man depend on the degree of closeness he has with the child and the length of time he interacts with it. Fathers who devotedly cared for their children have more oxytocin-secreting neurons in their brain, similar to mothers.

In a follow-up, Professor Feldman gave the fathers a synthetic oxytocin via an inhaler. Participants who inhaled oxytocin showed a ten-fold increase in the level of the hormone measured in their saliva. The level of oxytocin also increased in the babies' saliva and the change in the fathers' behaviour was noticeable. The fathers played twice as much with their children, looked into their eyes for longer, touched them more often and the babies cried less.

Professor Feldman and her research team also followed gay couples parenting adopted children. They arrived at the homes of the families and measured the oxytocin levels in the blood of the fathers and the babies. They found, of course, that the mechanism works exactly the same in these parents as well. The level of oxytocin increased and was very high during periods of parental caregiving. Moreover, the same triangular relationship was observed between the primary caregiver, who spends more time with the infant, the secondary caregiver and the baby, just like that found in the heterosexual couples.

The Effect of Babies on Their Fathers' Brains

As we have seen, the length of time it takes for a father to bond with his baby depends on the level of their physical and emotional interactions. Usually, in the first weeks and months of a newborn's life, the father's level of attachment is low compared to the mother's, due to the different amount of time they spend interacting with the baby. An experiment conducted at the University of Michigan examined how the brains of fathers and mothers react to the sound of their new baby crying, compared to the cries of other babies. They found that at first the father's brain does not respond to his baby's cries as quickly as the mother's brain does. However, after four weeks or so, the gap narrows and the father's reactions are similar to the mother's reactions to the baby's cry.

Fathers say that when you become a father you really feel like something has happened to your brain. No matter where you are or what you are doing, you feel a sense of alertness and vigilance toward your offspring. And while you care for and feed your baby, you are aware of every expression of emotion on their little face, every hiccup or sound of crying.

Indeed, when researchers from the universities of Denver and Yale scanned the brains of 16 new fathers about three weeks after the birth of their child and again at 15 weeks, they saw an increase in the volume of grey matter in the areas responsible for processing sensory information, similar to the increase in the brains of new mothers. An increase was also found in the area involved in attachment and nurturing in the fathers' brains. In addition, a decrease in the volume of grey matter was observed in parts of the brain associated with "autopilot" mode, the parts that are activated when we disconnect from the outside world. It is possible that the contraction of these areas reflects the renewed allocation of resources in favour of promoting vigilance toward the offspring. Another area that shrank as the father spent more time with his children was a part of the brain associated with feelings of anxiety.

Fathers also have moments of despondency, excessive irritability and stress, similar to mothers. Between 4 and 10 per cent of new fathers experience a clinical state of depression. The signs of postpartum depression in men are restlessness, anger, over-irritability, plunging into work for longer hours and increased alcohol consumption. Moreover, the father's risk level of experiencing postpartum depression increases if his partner also experiences postpartum depression. Other factors that may increase the risk are pressure at work, prolonged lack of sleep, the birth of twins or crises in marital relationships. Fathers who experience postpartum depression will interact less with the baby.

Similarly to fathers, adoptive mothers experience the same hormonal and neuronal changes as biological mothers, and bond with their children through the oxytocin mechanism, even without the process of pregnancy and birth. A hormonal mechanism works in such a way that the more the hormone is produced, the more receptors for it are created in the brain and the attachment gets tighter. The process of parenting in itself causes such an increased secretion of oxytocin and the hormones that accompany it, and changes the minds of parents for ever.

Parenting Passion Killers

Statistics show that relationship crises usually start to occur three years after the arrival of the first child, and then recur every five to seven years in a major meltdown. If you make it through the first five years, the more likely you are to sail calmly through the following years.

When we understand the magnitude and intensity of the changes that the mind and body go through in the transition to parenthood, along with the hormonal differences between mothers and fathers, the way the hormones work and the evolutionary logic in all this, it's not surprising that many couples report damage to their relationship and a decrease in intimacy after having children.

Our selfish genes rewire us to put the needs of the next generation before our own, to be attentive to them all the time, to feed them, lull them to sleep, clean, calm, nurture and protect them without fail. The main hormone that creates the drive to take care of our children's needs is prolactin. It is secreted into the blood from the pituitary gland in both mothers and fathers when they are with children. The smaller the child, the more prolactin is needed and the more is secreted.

When else is prolactin secreted? Immediately after orgasm, it produces a moment of calm, when we are not sexually responsive and experience a sharp decrease in sexual energy and a lack of desire. Prolactin also reduces the secretion of testosterone, which stimulates the sex drive.

Does this make evolutionary sense? Of course, as when there are children around, the energy of their parents should be directed to them. Children need parents who are emotionally stable, predictable and focused on them. They need security, certainty and routine – all factors that suppress eroticism and passion. (Erotica thrives precisely on conditions of uncertainty, insecurity and all that is unusual.) Therefore, being around young children increases the secretion of prolactin and decreases the secretion of testosterone and oestrogen. The end result is that sexual energy is switched off, and parental energy gets a boost.

In animals, while the mother is lactating and nursing, she will not be in heat. A female orangutan, for example, loses her libido for up to eight years as long as her offspring is with her. When the youngster leaves and she finds herself alone again, her sexual urge returns at once and she looks for a dominant male and woos him with renewed passion.

The other hormone besides prolactin that can slowly sabotage a couple's relationship, as their family expands, is cortisol, the stress hormone, the silent killer. Parenthood is accompanied by a dramatic increase in stress levels; a mother's cortisol level is often two to three times higher than before. Besides the many worries, concerns and anxieties about children and finances, this is a period characterized by a lack of sleep and continuous fatigue. Lack of sleep is a major source of stress, which affects all the mechanisms of our body, our mood and our general health. Fatigue, irritability, impatience and aggression are just some of the manifestations of a lack of sleep. Sleep disorders are a common phenomenon among young children and naturally cause sleep disorders in their parents. And just when the battle for sleep is coming to an end, when the first child starts sleeping through the night, a second child may be on the way and everything starts again. Therefore, it's not surprising that the parents of small children are the group that has the least sex.

Cortisol also suppresses the sex drive, as in times of stress the priority is not to waste energy on reproduction but to focus on survival. As we have seen, survival mode leads to the following options: fight, run away, freeze or tend and befriend. In the case of new parents, this can manifest itself in the following ways:

Fight: attacking your partner, blame them for all your troubles and nag them.

Escape: finding an escape hatch by spending more time at work, gazing at screens (television, telephone), fleeing to friends, playing excessive sports, alcohol, emotional eating, watching porn, looking for sex elsewhere, or using mind-numbing substances.

Freeze: sinking into depression, exhaustion, helplessness, a lack of motivation, energy and liveliness, too much sleep and shutting down.

Tend and befriend: taking care of the needs of others in an obsessive way. In this way, a vicious cycle is created – more stress leads to less contact, less intimacy and more trying to escape, so more feelings of guilt, more stress, less contact, less intimacy and so on . . . until the result is complete emotional detachment. We can also add to this cycle the Coolidge effect (see chapter 6, page 93) – the wiring that destroys desire, based on dopamine, which is built into the brain. This entails a decrease of excitement for the same partner and also of sensitivity to familiar stimulus as time goes by, and is a sure route to creating distance between a couple that can last for years, with or without any excitement sought on the side.

It is estimated that over 80 per cent of all women will experience a lack of attraction toward their partner during their life together that lasts for a period of over three months. About 60 per cent are not attracted to their partner for a period of six months, and about 20 per cent of all women – one in five – lose their passion for their partner for as long as one year. Some lose their libido altogether, and others experience a decrease in their sexual desire toward their partner but are still attracted to other men.

A decrease in libido is common mainly in women after the age of 30 – the time of motherhood, and after the age of 60 – post-menopause. These two periods of life are characterized by hormonal changes, increased stress and a decrease in sex hormones.

What about the libido of fathers? In 18 per cent of men, there is a loss of sexual desire toward their partner. The reasons for this can range from stress, anxiety, depression and a drop in testosterone that also results from fatherhood and later from the male menopause. From the age of 55, a man's testosterone level drops to a fifth of that of a young man.

Nevertheless, surveys point to a six-fold difference on average in the desire to have sex between men and women in committed relationships. Men want more and feel less satisfied. As previously mentioned, the male reproductive system differs from that of the female; men think more often about sex and need sexual contact in order to find release from stress and relax. A man whose partner suddenly loses all sexual interest in him often feels rejected and unloved, which will lead to increased tension in the relationship and the search for escape into work, sports, chemicals or friends. Men's primary love language is touch, whereas a woman's is language – empathy. Men need touch to relax and connect, women need words and empathy first. The reason for this is, of course, testosterone and oestrogen.

Research by Professor David Buss in the USA found that over 80 per cent of those married women surveyed had been asked by their spouse to have sexual relations during their married life for a number of reasons that were unrelated to their own desire or enjoyment of sex. When sex is not a freely chosen source of pleasure but becomes a chore, another item on a list of things needed from her at home, it too becomes much more of a stress factor than a calming factor or an erotic trigger.

Over time, a two-way mutual resentment may develop between the person who thinks they are doing a favour and the one who feels they are being done a favour. As we saw previously, 95 per cent of the communication between us is not verbal but takes place through expressing our feelings in our eyes, facial expressions, voice and, of course, body language. There is no place where nonverbal emotional communication is as strong as during sexual activity, where only the body speaks – and the body does not lie. We feel it in our stomachs. Within 15 milliseconds, our nervous system detects whether the other party is attracted and enjoying the touch or not. The seeds of tomorrow's fight are potentially sown the evening before in the bedroom during this nonverbal emotional communication between the couple.

Over time, the resentment may increase and the contact will decrease. This even has a name in the world of couples' therapy, "touchy aridity", a phenomenon that sooner or later will lead to the end of the relationship. We saw earlier how the release during physical contact of the love hormone, oxytocin, activates our vagus nerve, which rules our relaxation system, encouraging us to rest and digest. Our nervous system needs touch and connection to relax and feel safe. Lack of contact, and lack of relaxation, will cause an increase in stress, resentment and tension; hence the predictable path to emotional disconnection.

The Repression System and Parenting Under Pressure

Couples can stay together yet be emotionally distant for years – from decades to the rest of their lives.

When starting a family, the framework of marriage traditionally constitutes the social, emotional and economic infrastructure of that family's structure. Sex is a means of achieving family and family is the pillar of our mental wellbeing as human beings. We don't live in couples; we live in families, and our survival depends on our belonging to a social system from the moment we are born.

When we have children of our own, we are, as mentioned, programmed to protect, care for and take care of the minds and bodies of those children; we therefore usually find it relatively easy to put our own needs aside, as the main thing is to protect our children's lives. The connections we build with our children, and their love for us, are critical to our wellbeing – and a lot has to happen for us to allow damage to affect these connections.

In addition, our familial connections also play a role; for example, what will our parents, brothers or sisters think of us if we harm our family? A family is a multigenerational system whose members have the strongest influence on each other. To ensure our survival as part of the family system, one of the most powerful mechanisms of the human brain comes into play. It's been called the repression mechanism, which Freud referred to as being one of the most important defence mechanisms of the human brain. It's designed to prevent us from acting on impulse and endangering our survival.

Within our relationship with our partner, we therefore strive to repress any feelings, events or thoughts that could provoke a conflict and endanger the stability of that connection. We avoid "rocking the boat". Repression actually enables the maintenance of a reasonable marital relationship, at least outwardly. But over time, silencing and covering up their feelings can increase the distance and emotional disconnection between a couple. With the passing months and years, the list of topics to be avoided grows and conversations between the couple become increasingly tense with the effort of avoiding talking about the elephant in the room. The exchange becomes largely devoid of emotions and the "permitted" topics of conversation become ever more boring and technical.

Is there any difference between men and women regarding repression and denial? To one degree or another, both sexes use these defence mechanisms very effectively to maintain the status quo and support a *modus vivendi* – an agreement that allows us to coexist peacefully. However, men feel more uncomfortable talking about unpleasant feelings, and find it more difficult to explain in words what they feel or need from their partner. According to Dr John Gottman's research on quarrels between spouses, a strategy of stonewalling during a quarrel – disconnection and indifference – was about

80 per cent more common among men. When the men felt emotionally overwhelmed during the quarrel, they broke off contact. This is classic repression: avoiding dealing with unpleasant feelings.

Women experience this strategy as the most offensive and disrespectful, interpreting it as blatantly ignoring and dismissing their own feelings and needs. It leaves no room in which to release tension, or for reconciliation and empathy – and from their perspective the whole purpose of the quarrel may be about reconciliation. When women offer to try therapy and get help, men in the majority of cases will express a lack of interest. The common excuses for this are: *It's a waste of time and money*; *We don't need help, everything is fine*; and *What do therapists know? It's all nonsense.*

Naturally, the reason for this is testosterone inhibiting the areas of communication and empathy in the male brain, thereby increasing their self-confidence and creating an obsession with status; meaning that they will go all out in order not to show weakness and neediness. In addition to the effects of their biology, in a patriarchal society boys are educated to keep their feelings to themselves, not to show weakness outwardly and not to cry, but to withstand pressure and in principle not to be girlish.

The end result is a time lag between the onset of a crisis in the relationship and the couple seeking therapy. This takes six years on average, or, if you like, when the woman threatens a final breakup. (The majority of divorce proceedings in the world are initiated by women.) Six years of repressing negative feelings have turned into anger. Cortisol has accumulated into rivers of resentment, loathing, suppressed rage and even hatred bubbling under the surface, so that emotional reconnection will be difficult and in some cases impossible.

It is important to understand that when the couple or partner raises the need for therapy, they are saying in a roundabout way: "I am full of negative emotions, I feel distant and am longing for healing and connection." Ignoring these feelings through suppression and denial will activate the self-destruction mechanism of the relationship and it is only a matter of time until they disconnect emotionally, with or without physical separation.

So how does one preserve long-term love within the framework of a family? First of all by understanding how biology changes us when we become parents. Understand that focusing on care, concern and support for the offspring allows us to reduce slightly the frustration and guilt both men and women go through. A family is a connected neuronal unit. What happens in the minds of the children affects the parents, and what happens in the minds of the parents also affects the children. The stress level of the children affects the stress level of the parents and, of course, impacts the conjugal relationship.

As mentioned, children need stability, routine and certainty – parents are mostly boring and predictable and therefore the hormones in charge of nurturing turn off eroticism and passion. On the other hand, the emotional connection between the parents is also critical for the wellbeing of their children. When their parents are connected and loving, this calms a child's nervous system. The emotional connection between the parents also depends on the level of sexual satisfaction. So how can we resolve the paradox? This is a delicate balancing act and it depends on tuning into each other and awareness. If I am a mother of two children, who have many needs and difficulties, I may have to wait for sexual desire to reappear and I may have to wait for a long time. I can blame the fact on my partner, who "doesn't do it for me", but it's really nothing to do with him, it's all about biology; the Coolidge effect (see page 93) plus the stress of motherhood doesn't leave much chance for my sex drive. What is sad is that touch is so very important to reduce stress, yet there is no desire for touch in my stressful state. I might enter a vicious cycle of stress . . .

Therefore, taking responsibility for our sexuality is a necessity for us as parents. We need to embark on a journey of exploration and self-learning fuelled by curiosity. Buddhists say emotion is like a feather on a wall: one moment the wind moves it to the right of the wall, and the next moment the wind moves it to the other side. At the end of the day, the initial feeling is that there is no desire, but any action we take in that direction, such as a relaxing conversation, an enjoyable massage, being caressed, or watching an erotic video or playing with a sex toy together, will arouse desire. Sex should become something you do for you and not for your partner – we need touch and orgasms as much as possible to reduce stress and sleep better.

Let's not forget that at the end of the journey of raising children, menopause awaits us (for both women and men), which brings with it yet more hormonal changes and stress to the body. As mentioned, studies show that women who are more sexually active around menopause suffer from far fewer symptoms. It is important to understand that orgasms are a gift to the mind and body, no less than physical activity, a healthy diet and mindfulness.

Additional tools for preserving marital love can be found later in this book, including a scientifically based prescription for preserving long-term love in a challenging era.

CHAPTER 6
ARE WE PROGRAMMED FOR FIDELITY?

We have seen how, at the beginning of a relationship, the chemicals of love produce the experience of powerful infatuation and intense desire, with all the side effects that come with this. Unfortunately, however, this passion usually doesn't last long . . .

Sometimes, it can seem like there is a spell cast over long-term relationships: they start with intense passion, falling in love and longing; then, at some point, we move in together or decide to get married and are convinced that our love will last for ever. But within two to three years, a strange tension begins to arise; suddenly we feel that we need personal space in the relationship, our sexual attraction and desire decrease and doubts begin to arise regarding our partner. At this point, either we can stay together despite the doubts, or we can break up and start this whole dance again with someone new. Why do many relationships seem to follow a similar pattern? What exactly is that pattern, and is there a biological explanation for it?

If we were to draw an imaginary graph charting the intensity of excitement and desire toward a particular partner over time, which might be on a scale of months or years, it would appear that at the beginning of the relationship, when all stimuli are new, the intensity of excitement increases exponentially; that is, it takes off at an increasing rate. This period of time is defined as the "falling in love" phase; it's when you want to be together, touch all the time, and you miss each other when apart, experiencing withdrawal symptoms after a long separation, such as depression, irritability, lack of sleep and lack of appetite.

This period of falling in love can last from six hours to two years, but on average it's around a year. During the falling in love phase, when the oxytocin relationship has sufficiently solidified, we may move into the commitment phase, seeking to formalize the relationship and be together on a regular basis. Usually, a couple will decide to move in together, get married, give birth to a common child or unite their existing families if this is a second time around for them both.

During the commitment period, the desire and excitement graph straightens out; that is, the increase in excitement stops and stabilizes at a certain level. As time passes, the period of falling in love ends and is replaced by regular patterns of intimacy and routine. Over the years, and sometimes on a shorter time scale, a moderate dip in the graph of excitement and desire may appear. This decrease is characterized by a slow emotional and physical distancing, which is accompanied by a drying up of physical contact and sexuality, and which may lead to a sharp decrease in intimacy.

This phase on the graph marks the period of a relationship "at risk", since it is characterized by a sharp drop in joint oxytocin production. After all, if the relationship between two people who were complete strangers to each other until a few years or months ago is entirely the result of their joint production of oxytocin, as soon as they stop producing this hormone together – i.e., talk less, listen less, share less, touch each other less, kiss less, experience fewer joint orgasms – there is a high risk that the marital relationship will break up and the couple will return to being two strangers.

According to a survey conducted in Israel on the occasion of Family Day 2020, a national event, it was found that a third of married couples only communicate via WhatsApp. Needless to say, WhatsApp does not produce oxytocin at a significant level. Another survey found that only a tenth of married couples in Israel report satisfactory intimate relations. This data goes some way toward explaining the divorce data, which stands at one couple out of two in the secular Jewish population and one couple out of three in the general population in Israel, and one couple out of two on average in Western countries. The more developed the country, the higher the divorce rate.

In our modern era, which is freer from the restrictions and dictates of religion and culture, any institutionalized marital system has a 50 per cent chance of falling apart, with the chances of divorce being highest during the first five years of marriage. Every additional five years you stay together increases the chances of your making it through the next five years.

As we saw in chapter 5, according to the statistics, most of the crises experienced by married couples globally begin three years after the arrival of their first child. Some say it is the result of "routine" or "wear and tear", but we already understand that hormones, chemicals and neurons play an important role here. So what happens to love over time, and why does the graph of excitement and passion dwindle away? And if these phenomena are so universal, is it time to stop and ask if our brains are programmed, from an evolutionary point of view, to be excited and love the same person all our lives?

Without a doubt, the most disappointing side effect of the love chemicals is the phenomenon of tolerance – the decline. As you spend more time together, your partner becomes more and more familiar, the stimuli he or she provides are no longer new and the levels of dopamine and serotonin released in your brain in response to your partner decrease. The reward system, the dopamine system in the brain, loves novelty and variety. Everything bores us over time. The system turns on more strongly when it receives a new signal. When the same familiar signals are repeatedly received, the system's excitement threshold rises and the brain seeks variety.

Our excitement for the same partner decreases due to this tolerance, but returns in all its glory when presented with someone new. The effect that causes a decrease in sexual excitement with a regular partner and an increase in sexual excitement with a new partner is called the Coolidge effect, or the sexual saturation effect, and it exists in almost all mammals. We have touched upon the Coolidge effect earlier in this book, and it's very important to familiarize ourselves with this ancient and powerful wiring that evolution has embedded in our brains, which is responsible for at least half of the broken hearts in the world.

The Coolidge Effect

In the 1950s, researchers Frank Beach and Lisbeth Jordan at the University of Berkeley in the USA conducted a fascinating study on the sexual excitement of male rats. During a series of experiments, they placed a female rat in heat in a cage with a male rat and measured how long it took the male to ejaculate. At the start of the experiment, the male was presented with the same female rat each time. Female rats mate every four days, so every four days they popped her back in the male's cage. (The female underwent a procedure that prevented her from becoming pregnant so that she would continue to be amenable to fertilization.) However, in the second part of the experiment, two weeks later, they introduced a different female to the male every four days and made the same measurement.

The results were amazing. In the first experiment with the same female, each time the male mated with her it took him longer and longer to ejaculate.

The first time it took him two minutes (the average time for a male rat to reach orgasm is between two and four minutes). The second time he mated with her it took him three minutes, the third time five minutes, the fourth time it took him a quarter of an hour to achieve his goal, while the fifth time took seventeen minutes and on their eighth and ninth encounters he no longer approached her and didn't even try to mate with her.

However, in the second experiment, when a new female was presented to him every four days, our energetic lover maintained an average of two to three minutes to ejaculate and continued until exhaustion, even unto death, as long as new females were brought to him. The reason the rat died of exhaustion is that every time he met a new female, he increased the amount of sperm he ejaculated into her, and the production of sperm requires a huge amount of energy from the body.

The phenomenon of sexual saturation has been observed not only in male rats but also in the males of a variety of different mammals. But why does this phenomenon occur in the first place? Why does the male ejaculate faster with new females and slower and slower with the same female? The answer lies hidden in the emotional brain, in the dopamine system. The male's brain releases a higher level of dopamine before and during orgasm with a new female and a lower level of dopamine with a female he has already been exposed to.

In answer to why the male brain is programmed so that mating with a new female is more rewarding than with a familiar female, it is the reward for spreading his seed. The brain is programmed by the genes, and the male's genes reward him for spreading his sperm to as many females as possible, who will carry them into future generations. From the point of view of the genes, it makes no sense to mate every time with the same female in the wild, since hopefully she has already conceived the first time round and continuing to mate with her would be a waste of time. Male rats do not share in raising their offspring; like 97 per cent of mammals, they are polygamous creatures and are kept busy by fighting other males and fertilizing females. In polygamist structures, the males do not bond with one female but try to impregnate as many females as possible during their lifetime.

After continuing the experiments and repeatedly seeing the sexual satiety effect in the males, the researchers at Berkley wanted to understand how the signal reaches the male's brain. How does he differentiate between the new female and the familiar one? In an attempt to answer this question, they smeared vaginal secretions from a new female rat onto the skin of a familiar female. In this situation, when she was covered with the vaginal secretions of the new female, the male took her to be new too and reached his climax very quickly. That is, the signal was sent to the dopamine system in his brain through the smell of the pheromones found in the vaginal secretions. He identified and differentiated between the females according to the pheromone smell unique to each one.

The sexual saturation effect, as mentioned, is very strong and it has also been found in stallions, male donkeys, roosters, chimpanzees and other animals. This wiring, which encourages males to mate with as many females as possible, has tremendous value for genes, which wish to ensure the greatest number of copies in the next generation, and has therefore endured throughout evolution. Why, then, did it get the popular name the "Coolidge effect"?

Coolidge was not the scientist who discovered the phenomenon, but the name of the 30th President of the United States, Calvin Coolidge, to whom a famous anecdote is attributed. During his presidency he accompanied Grace, his wife of 25 years, on a visit to a farm in Texas to see the new advances in chicken farming. Grace entered one of the chicken coops and when the farmer told her about the various innovations, the First Lady was more interested in the fact that you don't need more than one rooster in a flock with 20 to 30 hens. Impressed by the bird's virility, Grace politely said to the farmer, "Tell that to the President when he comes by."

When Coolidge entered the coop, the embarrassed farmer said to him: "Mr President, your wife asked me to tell you about this rooster."

The President listened attentively and then asked the farmer, "Same hen every time?"

"Certainly not, sir," said the farmer. "A different hen each time."

"Then tell it to Mrs Coolidge," President replied.

Professor Frank Beach was aware of the story and decided to call the sexual saturation effect he discovered in males after the President.

Does the Coolidge Effect Work Both Ways?

So far we have talked about males. But what about females? Is the Coolidge effect evident in them as well? Do they prefer the new over the familiar, or do they prefer to mate with the same person over and over again?

In every lecture I gave, I put this question to the audience and most of the women chorused in unison, "I prefer the same one."

And I'd reply, "You're kidding yourselves."

Until one evening a woman said to me, "What do you expect me to answer? My husband is sitting right here next to me!"

More than 30 years passed before scientists decided to test whether the sexual saturation effect also exists in females (the delay being further evidence of scientific bias). In the late 1980s, researchers from the University of British Columbia in Canada took a virgin vole in heat and placed her in a large cage divided into three cells. The female was placed in the middle cell and, on either side, there were one-way openings from which she could pass to the neighbouring cells. Only the female could choose which cell she wanted to enter, and the entrance to her cell was blocked.

At the start of the experiment, the researchers placed a young male in the right-hand cell. The assumption was that since she was fertile the female would enter his cell, mate with him and bond with him thanks to the oxytocin released in their brains during orgasm. Following the process of attachment and falling in love, she was expected to return to him every few days for more satisfaction. In order to allow continued oestrus after mating, the researchers performed a procedure to prevent the female from becoming pregnant.

Simultaneously, every few days the researchers introduced an impressive new male into the left-hand cage and observed which cage the female visited more often. The first thing the researchers noticed was that, unlike the male, who immediately leaped into action, the female lingered and wasn't in a rush to go anywhere; she carefully examined, checked, compared and selected the males. Finally, the researchers saw that she did indeed return to the first male with whom she had previously mated, but occasionally examined the new male in the left-hand cage and mated with him as well, if he was interesting enough.

The researchers concluded that the Coolidge effect exists in females too, but is moderate compared to that in males. The female's mind also receives pleasure and reward from exposure to new stimulation, just like the male does, but since she bears the entire burden of pregnancy, birth, nursing and rearing the offspring, she is very calculating and selective when choosing her mating partners. If the effect is milder in females, there may be a connection between this and testosterone, since the testosterone level in females is lower. It is also possible that testosterone increases the Coolidge effect in males and acts on the reward mechanism – the release of dopamine that rewards them more for new stimuli than familiar stimuli. Proof that testosterone is responsible for the Coolidge effect was found in a study wherein it disappeared in castrated males, the testicles being the testosterone production factory.

Has a study been conducted that proves the existence of the Coolidge effect among women and not just in rats and voles? Not yet. It's known that women watch less porn than men. One hundred million people visit the PornHub website every day, and five million new videos are uploaded every year. Only about a quarter of the viewers are female and it is interesting to note, according to the website's data, that the most watched category among women depicts lesbians, and in second place is the category of threesomes. While the Coolidge effect has not yet been proven in human females, but to me, it would be very interesting to see what happens in a matriarchal society, in which women are dominant.

It's estimated that there is only one such society remaining in the world. The Muso tribe in northern China is a matriarchal society where inheritance, according to tradition, passes from grandmother to daughter to granddaughter. The women, especially the grandmothers, are the ones who manage the affairs of the community.

We might expect that in such a society, where women are dominant, every woman has a devoted, attentive and loyal husband waiting for her at home. But that is not the case in this tribe. In the Muso language, the words "father", "husband" and "marriage" do not exist. According to tradition, when a girl reaches maturity, she gets her own room and can choose to have a relationship with whomever she wants. The lucky man comes over in the evening, usually with something nice to eat or drink, they sleep together and in the morning he leaves and returns to his grandmother's house.

When a child is born, the identity of the biological father is irrelevant. The brothers and sisters help the daughter of the family to raise the child. Sometimes the women form a long-term relationship with the same partner for years. However, when she feels the relationship has run its course, according to tradition there is no "where are we going with this" conversation; instead, she hangs a red flag on the balcony. This is a sign for the man that the relationship is over, he packs his belongings and does not return. The red flag is also a sign to other men that she is now available.

The Muso tribe teach us that in a matriarchal society, there is no need for paternity verification. A woman and a man stay together only for the purpose of love and companionship and not in order to raise children and pass along an inheritance. It should be noted that from the moment the Muso community was exposed to the Western world and curious tourists began to arrive, the society changed and lost its matriarchal characteristics.

The Coolidge Effect and Our Sexual Fantasies

In 2001, researchers in Australia sat a group of young men in front of a screen showing a short porn video in a loop, repeating the same scene over and over again. While the men watched the video, the researchers tested their arousal physically, by measuring their erections, and in writing, by asking them to fill out a questionnaire. The researchers found that as the men watched the same video over and over again, their stimulation, both physical and mental, decreased. After watching the same video 19 times, when the men were almost falling asleep in front of the screen, the researchers replaced the scene with a video showing different actresses acting out the same plot. Miraculously, the men were immediately highly stimulated again, affecting both their erections and written reports.

This was scientific evidence of the Coolidge effect in the male human, involving a decrease in stimulation from a familiar signal and an increase in stimulation when presented with a new signal. With us, unlike rats and voles, the signal has less to do with smell – although pheromones still do play a role in our sexual stimulation – and more to do with the eyes. We are visual creatures; half of our brains are used for processing visual information, so visual images of new women are arousing. The billion-dollar porn industry relies heavily on the Coolidge effect and the need to continually produce new images, films and videos.

It is important to note that our brain, which developed on the savannas of Africa, has never been exposed to so many powerful sexual stimuli as it is today. When consuming porn, the dopamine system is flooded, leading to the phenomena of porn addiction and sex addiction. The brain then develops a tolerance to these stimuli, so that each time stronger and stronger signals are needed in order for an individual to reach orgasm. Increased porn consumption causes the viewer to increase the time spent watching it and to seek out ever more explicit content in order to reach the same levels of stimulation.

In a study in which the brain activity of men addicted to porn was examined in relation to an impairment of their social functioning, and then compared to the brain activity of cocaine addicts, the researchers noted the same areas of the reward system – the pleasure system – were lit up in the brains of the participants of both groups.

Porn reflects the sexual fantasies of humans, the sexual stimuli at work in our brains, and affords us a glimpse into our primal and ancient animal mind, unfettered by the social and moral inhibitions of the prefrontal cortex. What stimuli turn on our brains? And are we ready to talk about this openly and scientifically? Scientists are not keen to investigate such an explosive issue, which goes beyond the realms of social-political correctness. But there is one person who has studied sexual fantasies deeply, including the differences between the sexual fantasies of men and women. He is the American social psychologist Professor Roy Baumeister. In 2000, Baumeister published a study in which 1,500 women and men from different cultures around the world participated and were asked to describe in detail their most frequent sexual fantasies. Our fantasies may often seem highly personal and unique to us, but since we all belong to the same species – *Homo sapiens* – and were born with more or less the same brain, there are plenty of similarities shared by men and a different set of similarities common to women.

From an analysis of the research participants' answers, it was found that the most common fantasy of heterosexual men in all cultures of the world is, as expected, sex with two or more women, regardless of religion, colour, race or nationality. In other words, the Coolidge effect at its best, stimulating more powerful orgasms for real-time sperm distribution. The second most common fantasy, as reported by men from different cultures, was noncommittal sex. Again, the recurring motif is a multiplicity of partnerships – remember that the genes reward multiplicity with pleasure.

What, then, was the most common fantasy found among women from different cultures? As might be expected, the answer is not quite so simple and straightforward. It became clear from the data analysis that the most common fantasy of women depends largely on the society in which a woman lives. For women living in powerfully patriarchal societies, where men dominate women and women's status is low, the most common female fantasy was of a strong, controlling and dominant man. A significant percentage fantasized about forced sex. On the other hand, in women from more egalitarian societies where the status of women is generally higher, the most common fantasy was of exhibitionism: the woman imagines that several men and/or women are watching her as she pleasures herself or as she has intercourse.

The difference between the sexual fantasies of women in different societies caused the researcher to call the phenomenon "female erotic plasticity". As we can see, the Coolidge effect appears to play a role in both men's and women's fantasies. An image of multiple and diverse partners increases the level of dopamine in the brain during sexual stimulation. That's why sometimes during sex with their regular partner, many report that they fantasize about other people in order to reach a better orgasm.

These fantasies can often evoke feelings of shame and guilt, which is why it's important to understand the extent to which fantasizing is a biological and natural process related solely to the way our brains are wired by evolution – and not to something lacking in our partner or our relationship. The emotional, sexual brain is programmed to look for as many options as possible in order to diversify the genetic makeup of the next generation and is rewarded for this with dopamine and adrenaline, excitement and pleasure. It doesn't matter how perfect our relationship is or how good our partner is to us and to the kids, our brain is looking for the sort of primal thrills that we and most other mammals share.

A Question of Fidelity

Sometimes the longing for diversity does not remain at the level of fantasy, and people form casual or continuous sexual relationships with additional partners outside the framework of their permanent relationship. We call it betrayal or adultery, and it is the most common yet least discussed phenomenon among people in different societies around the world. When people were asked in anonymous surveys, "Have you ever cheated on your partner?" around half responded in the affirmative. When the question was altered to, "If it's guaranteed that you will never be caught, would you cheat?" 85 per cent answered yes.

The phenomenon is not unique to humans. Even animals that have just the one permanent mate, and which raise offspring together, often cheat and hide it from their partners. In an experiment conducted with pigeons, genetic tests were performed on the eggs in the nest and compared to the DNA of the brooding male. About a third of the eggs did not match his DNA.

The sexual saturation effect explains why after some time in a relationship people are willing to risk a lot to experience the thrill of dopamine-rich orgasms with new partners. If we look at the phenomenon of infidelity from an evolutionary point of view, it's a smart adaptation. On the one hand, you don't break the bond of your permanent pairing, which affords maximum security and support for any existing offspring. On the other, if you are a male and play away from time to time, hiding this from your partner, you give your brain a little wakeup call and spread some more of your genes.

If you are female, you collect some good genes from outside the relationship and don't put all your eggs in one basket.

Since the wiring of the Coolidge effect is so strong, society has created social prohibitions to prevent the dissolution of relationships and damage to the family structure. As most societies are patriarchal, the most severe prohibitions have been placed on women rather than men. In our modern era, with the weakening of religious institutions and the rise of the internet, new challenges have arisen for the human mind. Finding available partners is easier, the speed of our interactions has increased and so has our ability to hide them. In the virtual age, opportunities for pursuing sexual or emotional relationships with other people literally sit in the palm of your hand. Since jealousy has not yet been eradicated from our arsenal of emotions – because in evolutionary terms not enough time has passed – it's difficult for us to accept a reality in which our much loved partner enjoys loving relationships with others. This is why we find ourselves in a difficult era for relationships; our confidence level has dropped yet our mind is constantly flooded with stimuli.

CHAPTER 7

THE WINNER TAKES IT ALL

The Coolidge effect, or sexual saturation effect, encourages genetic distribution and diversity, and thus causes many different problems for couples around the world. It plays a significant part in breakups, divorces, betrayals, confusion and heartbreak. Our genes are not interested in our personal happiness. Our mission is to pass as many copies of them as possible on to the next generation, no matter the cost. That is what we are rewarded for.

In his book *The Selfish Gene*, Richard Dawkins was the first to propose the idea that we might actually be just "vehicles" that genes use to transmit themselves to the next generation: the hen is the egg's means of producing another egg. From this perspective, I would be a good gene machine if I were to give birth to four children from four different men and not four children from one man, because in doing so I give my genes four diverse options for survival. Various combinations of genes from four men increase the chances that any one of the children would survive in a changing environment.

The genes of both the female and the male want diversity, but there is only one machine that is capable of producing offspring and who therefore always knows for sure that a percentage of the genes are hers, and that is the female. It is estimated that between 10 and 15 per cent of people are not the biological children of the father who gace them their surname, according to DNA testing. Usually it is the oldest or the youngest child in a family. In other words, it is assumed that the mother was already pregnant at the beginning of the relationship or had an affair a few years in. Females, on the whole, know who they mate with, but males are doomed to perpetual uncertainty. This situation is the source of the war between the sexes and the root of patriarchy and the obsessive need of males for control and confirmation of paternity throughout the animal kingdom.

Males have developed two strategies to make sure their genes are passed on to the next generation. These strategies have proven to be effective and have survived over millions of years of evolution. The first strategy: spread your seed! At any given moment there are myriad chances you will be recognized by a predator because of your feathers or colours, or be shoved aside by males stronger than you, so take advantage of every opportunity and focus on finding fertile females with whom you can share your seed. In order to make sure you don't get confused and become too attached, testosterone will boost the Coolidge effect for you, making you seek new thrills with new females. Remember, all the testosterone-filled males around you also want to spread their sperm, so you have to be faster and smarter than them. Eliminate competitors from the environment, even if they are your sons who have reached the age of sexual maturity.

The second strategy: keep females on a short leash. Dominate them. Don't let them get too close to other males and don't let other males get close to them; that's the only way you can make sure the offspring are yours. If possible, combine the two strategies, create your own harem of females and dominate them with a firm hand – in other words, polygamy.

Presented with these situations, what is the most effective strategy for the female? She bears all the burden of pregnancy, giving birth and raising offspring. She is always certain that the children are hers. And all the males want her. In terms of genes, she should focus on choosing the best candidate and carefully consider which male seems to have the best seed. With the most successful genes from her surroundings, she can increase her offspring's own chances of survival. If she finds the best of all, she should stay with him; he will protect her and her offspring from other males.

The importance for females of choosing the best can be seen in cheetahs and some other felines, who do not ovulate until they witness a sprinting competition between the males. Watching the males run is the signal their ovaries need to ovulate. After watching the running competition, they all want the winner. He is the fastest, the strongest, the biggest, the most beautiful, the most muscular, the bravest, or, depending on the species, the one who sings the most beautifully – depending on what she is looking for, as long as he is an alpha male or as close to an alpha as possible.

In vervet monkeys, for example, when a fight breaks out between neighbouring groups, the females observe with great interest the degree of courage shown by the males from their group during the conflict. In the midst of the fighting, those males who didn't show bravery in battle, but were afraid and hid, receive a cold shoulder and even a scolding and a slap from the females. Conversely, males who have shown courage receive more attention and the females are more responsive to having sex with them. There is a tremendous amount of pressure on the male of a species. If you don't prove yourself, your chances of passing on your genes to the next generation diminish. Therefore, the males fight – and the winner takes all. Everyone makes room for the alpha male, giving him privileges over both females and territory.

The Triumph of the Alpha Male

The reward for triumphing over other males is huge. This is why, in nature, males are mainly preoccupied with the struggle for social hierarchy. In chimpanzee societies, for example, a male attacks a male once every six hours; a male attacks a female, usually sexually, once every 13 hours; and a female attacks a female once every 100 hours. Among gorillas, when a male beats all the others, a silver stripe appears on his back. This is the silverback alpha. However, if he starts losing fights, the silver stripe disappears and appears on the back of the new winner, and the females usually leave the loser and go with the victor.

For males, it's important that females see the signs of their victory. This is called the testosterone winner effect. Every time a male wins a fight, the level of testosterone in his blood increases, which causes changes in his appearance – secondary sex signs. Every creature has its particular signs. In cattle, the horns will grow and become sharper, in birds, the feathers will become more colourful and impressive, while the muscle mass of the chimpanzee and gorilla will increase, and so on. The winning male will gain control over the territory, the resources and the breeding rights, and the females will follow him and stay with him as long as he is victorious.

The sexual arousal of females toward the large, strong and dominant male, combined with the primal ambition of all males to be the alpha, helps explain, from an evolutionary point of view, the prevalence of the coercive sex fantasy present in both women and men – "to be alpha and be with the alpha" – which has been confirmed by several studies. In 1974, the researchers Hariton and Singer found that "subduing or being subjugated" was the second most common fantasy in both sexes. In 1988, it was discovered that more than half of the women who participated in a survey had fantasies about forced sex. The explanation given for the prevalence of this compulsive fantasy in women, according to psychology, is that these are the mind's protective mechanisms, which allow women to deal with their fears through fantasies. That is, if a woman has a fear of rape, then she will experience it as an erotic fantasy as a way of dealing with that fear. This is one explanation, but if we could conduct the same surveys among chimpanzees, geese, chickens, cats and dogs, we might find that they also fantasize about forced sex. In nature, as previously mentioned, geese and other females lay eggs only when the male bites them on the neck and they feel their full weight pressing down on them.

As we have seen, our fantasies allow us a glimpse into our primitive animal sexual mind, where violence and sex are interconnected. Throughout the animal kingdom, violence and sex are mediated by the same hormone, testosterone, which produces the sex drive as well as the aggressive and obsessive drive for hierarchy. Because males are blessed with more generous doses of testosterone, they are more sexual and aggressive, and females are attracted to those displaying the traits of testosterone. Alpha males in nature are not gifted with hypersensitivity or excesses of empathy. On the contrary, they are often more narcissistic, obsessed with their status, and more aggressive toward both males and females. The forced sex fantasy is actually a testosterone fantasy, the longing we all have for the hormone of power and control.

When a new alpha male mammal comes to power, he often wastes no time in killing the young of the male that preceded him. As long as the females are lactating they will not ovulate, so the alpha male kills them. He wants the females to ovulate so he can pass his genes on in the little time he has before a new rival for the crown defeats him. The female will mourn her loss for a day or two, then ovulate due to the cessation of nursing, and go to the new alpha to be fertilized.

Females have developed different ways to deal with the brutal killing of their young every time a new alpha comes along. In some species, they retire to the edge of the territory, to the periphery, to raise their existing offspring quietly. In many mammals, the smell of the pheromones of a new male produces an abortion signal in pregnant females, which causes the termination of the pregnancy and reabsorption of the foetus in the mother's body. Before the ruler kills the offspring, the mother kills it. This phenomenon is called the Bruce effect (after the scientist Hilda Bruce) and its evolutionary logic is to stop the mother investing energy in the foetus, because when it is born the new alpha will kill it anyway. The experiment that proved the effect was performed on mice: when the urine of an adult male was placed in a cage of pregnant females, they aborted the embryos. The smell of pheromones triggers an increased secretion of cortisol, the stress hormone, which causes placental abruption. Some claim that the effect also exists in humans and causes some cases of spontaneous abortion that have no other explanation.

Wars between males continue at the level of sperm themselves. Have you ever wondered why 360 million sperm cells are needed to fertilize a single egg? The reason is that most sperm cells are simply not used for fertilization, but for all-out warfare in the womb. According to studies carried out by the biologist Dr Robin Baker, when spermatozoa enter the vagina, 20 per cent of them are the pioneers, swimming quickly toward the uterus in order to fertilize the egg. However, 40 per cent fight a rearguard action, settling in the cervix and clumping together like a cork to prevent new sperm from entering and interfering. The other 40 per cent are defenders: they contain a toxin at the end of the cell nucleus (the head) and they feed on any spermatozoa belonging to other males that are found in the uterus, sticking to them, injecting them with the toxin and eliminating them. A sort of kamikaze spermatozoa. Every sexual contact is war. You never know who was here before and which sperm might be in the uterus. For this reason, males, including humans, increase the number of sperm cells emitted during orgasm with a new, previously unknown female.

Survival of the Fittest . . . and Best Adapted

In recent years, scientists have started to understand more about the superpowers of sperm cells. In December 2014, scientists Brian Dias and Kerry Ressler from Emory University in Atlanta published a seminal article in the journal *Nature Neuroscience* in which they reported ground-breaking research in the field of genetics.

The researchers took male and female mice and conditioned their brains to associate the smell of vanilla (which is usually a neutral smell for mice) with an electric shock. Every time the vanilla scent was diffused in the cage, the floor of the cage was electrified. After several times, the mice formed a connection between the scent and the shock, and attempted to flee when they smelled vanilla. So far, so much classic conditioning.

In the next step, the researchers took the males and females that had been mated and paired them with males and females that had not been mated. Amazingly, the mated males passed on the new information to their offspring, and their offspring also ran away when they smelled vanilla in the cage, even though they had never experienced an electric shock and had never smelled the scent before. However, the mated females didn't pass this information on to their offspring, only the males did. It seems a male can bequeath new information he has acquired to his offspring through the sperm cells he produces. This means that acquired traits can be passed from generation to generation through sperm cells.

In the annals of the development of the theory of evolution, a fascinating debate is recorded between Charles Darwin and Jean-Baptiste Lamarck, a 19th-century French naturalist. Darwin claimed that parents couldn't pass on to their offspring traits that had been acquired during their lifetime, while Lamarck argued that it was possible. Their argument revolved around the question of why a giraffe has a long neck.

Darwin reasoned that in the beginning there had been giraffes with short necks and a few with slightly longer necks; then there was a change in the environment and there were more leaves on the tops of the trees, as a result of which the giraffes with short necks died and only those with the long necks remained. However, Lamarck argued that in every generation the giraffes used their neck muscles to reach the fresh leaves on the treetops, and the trait was passed on to their offspring and thus the neck lengthened. Dias and Ressler's research proves that Lamarck was right, and in a big way, since it shows that fathers pass on to their offspring traits they've acquired during their own lifetime, traits that are useful for survival.

In their next step, Dias and Ressler wanted to understand what mechanism transmits the information inside the sperm cells. It turns out that there are epigenetic changes in certain genes on the DNA inside the cells. Epigenetic changes are chemical changes that occur in the genes following stimuli from the environment, which cause a change in the expression of certain proteins in the cells. This complex process is called epigenetic paternal inheritance, and its discovery proves that evolution operates in much more diverse ways than previously thought. This means of paternal inheritance reinforces the evolutionary logic behind the females' selection of alpha males, who have the most successful genes for coping with their given environment. The female wants to pass on these traits to her offspring. Therefore, she wants the male to be at his peak – experienced, strong, brave and unafraid to take risks – and bring in new information from that environment.

What Role Do Males Really Play?

Perhaps this epigenetic mechanism provides the explanation for one of the greatest mysteries of evolution: why were males created in the first place?

Biologists find it difficult to explain why sexual reproduction involving males and females – which requires a lot of resources for searching out a partner, having sex, and so on – is highly developed, while asexual reproduction, when only females reproduce without the need for males (called parthenogenesis) has been less successful. This is despite the fact that asexual reproduction is more economical in resources and produces more copies faster.

Among plants, insects, molluscs, fish, reptiles and even birds there is still a degree of possibility that reproduction can take place without sperm. For example, under certain conditions, when there is no sperm present, the DNA in an egg can duplicate itself and a chick is born that only has a mother, no father. However, from an evolutionary point of view, such duplications are not as beneficial, because when all the children are duplicates of the mother there will be insufficient genetic diversity. So when a change in the environment occurs – for example, if a new virus emerges – all the offspring may die.

In contrast, snails and worms get along fine as bisexuals, having both a uterus and eggs and sperm. If a snail meets another snail, they shove their "love sticks" into each other (usually a violent act), transfer sperm to each other, and store it for lonely times ahead. This means that if you're a snail and you don't encounter any other snails, you can still produce offspring from your eggs alone.

Among ants and bees, the queen lays eggs from which mostly female workers hatch, while a very few males will emerge from unfertilized eggs. These males have no father, only a mother. They live only until the wedding night of their mother queen, when they fly through the air in a wedding dance, violate their mother and immediately drop dead on the floor. Inside the cells of the males there is only one copy of each chromosome instead of two copies – half the number of chromosomes of their sisters. That is because their primary role is to screen defective genes from the colony.

Why is this? Because if each male has only one copy of each chromosome, then a male that has successfully hatched proves that he has completed his embryonic development normally and has a normal set of chromosomes. If there had been a mutation in one of the genes on the chromosomes, he would not have been born. Thus, through the males, the colony removes from the system any genes that have accumulated mutations.

In giant tube worms, the male is more or less a small testicle that drifts in the sea hoping to find a female. The female worm is huge and has an opening near the uterus that is ready and willing to receive these drifting testicles – you could call it a sac full of husbands. She then carries her males inside her and fertilizes herself with their seed as and when she sees fit.

Among mammals, the male has evolved to be the king of animals; large, muscular, standing up to danger and imposing terror (theoretically). This may have come about because mammals changed their reproductive strategy from quantity to quality: fewer offspring who receive maximum parental investment, instead of millions of offspring with minimal investment. Fewer offspring means a greater risk of losing all the investment in the next generation in the event of unexpected changes in the environment; therefore there is a need for constant gene improvement through the struggles of the males and the continuous transfer of the best genetic improvements, favouring the victorious high-status males.

This being the case, then the most reliable reproductive strategy from an evolutionary standpoint, and the one that has proven to be the most efficient for both female and male genes, is polygamy. The winner takes all. The warring males compete, and only one emerges victorious and gets all the privileges of territory and females. The females are all attracted to him, mate with him, raise only his offspring and stay with him until he is defeated by someone younger and stronger. The strategy is so stable that 95 per cent of creatures in nature are patriarchal polygamists.

However, one mammal in nature is matriarchal, and that is the hyena. The hyenas have an alpha female but not an alpha male. In hyenas the system is reversed, as the females have a higher testosterone level than the males. Hyena females are incredibly strong and large, and their genitals are almost exactly the same as those of the male. The clitoris is as prominent and erect as the male genital organ. In addition, females have a scrotum similar to that of a male, except that these sacs are filled with fibrous tissue. Regarding the social order, it is interesting to see that among the hyenas, after the hunt, the females let their offspring eat first, then other females according to their hierarchical status, and finally males get the leftovers. In patriarchal mammals, the males eat first according to their rank, then the females, also according to their rank, and finally the offspring.

Which group do we humans belong to? To the polygamous species (without doubt, patriarchal) or to the monogamous species? To answer this question, we must take a closer look at what monogamy is and when it developed. We need to familiarize ourselves with monogamous species and understand what is special about them compared to the rest of the animal kingdom.

CHAPTER 8
ARE HUMANS NATURALLY MONOGAMOUS?

Monogamy is a pattern of behaviour in which one female and one male create an exclusive long-term relationship, remain faithful to each other and jointly raise their offspring. About 5 per cent of species in nature are monogamous.

Penguins, pigeons, arctic wolves, cichlid fish, prairie voles, marmoset monkeys, gibbons and porcupines are all on the list. Most monogamous species live in a challenging environment, facing periodic food shortages or harsh climates, an abundance of predators or, like birds, must fly over huge areas looking for food. What all monogamous have in common is that in order to bring back food, someone must look after the offspring. That is, both a mother and a father are needed to take care of them. When the mother flies out of the nest to look for food, the father protects the eggs, which are of great nutritional value and are therefore at risk from predators. Then they switch roles: Mum looks after the nest while Dad looks for food.

If the environmental conditions allow a mother to manage raising the offspring on her own, monogamy will not develop in a species, because polygamy is more efficient in terms of genes. However, in an environment where mothers cannot fend for themselves and their eggs or cubs are constantly being eaten by predators, a change takes place. Then there is an advantage to having fathers stay and take care of their offspring, bonding in a stable pairing with one female, the mother of their young, and not pursuing other females. In such circumstances, individuals in these pairings survive longer and pass on their genes to the next generation along with a preference for monogamy, and thus monogamy develops in some species.

The Coolidge effect is weaker for monogamous males and females. They experience more sexual arousal and sexual excitement with the same partner than with someone new. But what happens when you finish raising your offspring and the chicks leave the nest? Do you stay together? It turns out not to be the case. At the end of the breeding season, the vast majority of the pairings in a monogamous species separate and look for a new mate. They don't stay together for life but change partners each breeding season. We call these serial monogamists, or social monogamists. But why break up after the breeding season rather than stay together for life? Of course, the answer has once again to do with our programmers, the genes, who are constantly pushing us to diversify partners.

Have you raised offspring that can go on to reproduce on their own? Excellent! Now is the time to diversify, and look for your own new partners. Moreover, in order not to waste any opportunity to mix with good genes, even while raising offspring, the monogamous cheat at every opportunity. As we have seen, a third of the chicks in a pigeon's nest don't belong to the brooding male. So the next time you compare a couple to "a pair of love birds", think twice. A more appropriate comparison might be "like a pair of albatross", because the albatross is the most monogamous creature in nature.

Among monogamous species, there is a subgroup of about a dozen that remain faithful to each other for their entire lives and never separate. These species are called "genetically monogamous" or "sexually monogamous". For genetic monogamists, the Coolidge effect does not exist at all, and they get excited every time by the touch of the same partner for the whole of their lives together. Among the dozen or so genetically monogamous creatures in the animal kingdom, we find the albatross, the mute swan, the cichlid fish, the short-tailed grouse, the Malaysian rat, the black eagle, the lar gibbon and the prairie warbler. A handful of species out of eight million means the probability of finding "eternal love" on Earth is 1 in 667,000 or a 0.17 per cent chance. The mathematics of love seem to be getting more and more depressing by the minute.

The Genetics of Monogamy

What is different about the biology of these genetic monogamists compared to everyone else? Is there a monogamy gene? In 2016, Dr Larry Young and his partners at the Center for Behavioral Neurobiology at Emory University in Atlanta published a fascinating study that sheds light on the genetics of monogamy. The researchers made a comparison between the brain and the genome (the entire DNA sequence) of prairie voles, which are genetically monogamous, and the genome and the brain of their close cousins, the meadow voles, which are completely polygamous, like most voles and rodents. Using this comparison, the researchers sought to understand the biological mechanisms of monogamy.

Prairie voles are small rodents found in the central United States and Canada, often in urban areas where there are many predators, so it is necessary for them to be alert all the time. They maintain strong and stable relationships throughout their lives and do not change partners at the end of the breeding season. The male prairie vole behaves very differently from his cousins, the male meadow voles. He becomes attached to the first female he meets immediately after his first orgasm and does not leave her for the rest of his life. If the female is taken away from him he sinks into depression and will shun food until she returns. He likes to rub up against her and snuggle with her at every opportunity. The Coolidge effect takes no hold on him and he therefore never tires of his chosen partner. Even when she dies he doesn't go looking for someone else. The prairie vole is unusually dedicated to taking care of his offspring every breeding season; by all accounts the perfect husband and father. So what creates this prince of the prairies? (And how do you make one?)

First of all, the researchers compared the genomes, the total DNA sequence, of the monogamous urban prairie vole to that of its cousin, the polygamous meadow vole, which inhabits grasslands in an environment with relatively few predators and plenty of food. Let's look at the differences between the city boy and his country cousin. There is a variance between them in the control region of one particular gene, the gene that codes the creation of receptors for the hormone vasopressin, the male version of oxytocin, the love hormone. Vasopressin, like oxytocin, is responsible for attachment and bonding. It is also responsible for territorial behaviour and defending offspring. The control region of a gene is responsible for the strength of the expression of that gene; that is, how much protein will be produced from it in a certain cell. It turns out that in the urban voles, a change occurred over time in the control region of the gene for the vasopressin receptor which has caused a higher expression of receptors for the love hormone, and it is this that completely transforms the prairie vole's behaviour.

When the researchers examined the brains of the prairie voles, compared to the meadow voles, they found that the monogamous prairie voles have more receptors for the love hormone on neurons, nerve cells, in the pleasure and reward system of the brain. Similar expressions of multiple receptors for the love hormone in the "pleasure and reward" system are found in the brains of mother prairie voles. That is to say, the mind of a monogamous vole father becomes similar to that of a vole mother as far as the mechanisms of love and attachment are concerned. Both bond with their offspring and with each other, and take devoted care of their family and enjoy it. The testosterone level of the monogamous prairie vole is low, and he is more similar in appearance and behaviour too to the female.

In their next step, Dr Young and his team had to prove that this change in the vasopressin receptor gene, which they named the "monogamy gene", is what causes the male prairie vole to be monogamous and behave the way it does. To do this, the researchers had to use genetic engineering to change the control area of the gene in a polygamous meadow vole. Amazingly, as a result of this change, the polygamous meadow vole also became monogamous; its brain was altered and it exhibited monogamous behaviour just like its cousin the prairie vole did.

This was a seminal study, showing how a change in the gene causes a change in the brain that leads to a change in behaviour, and so it was deduced that monogamy has a strong genetic basis. In nature, this change happens over time due to changing environmental conditions. In the challenging surroundings in which the prairie voles live, monogamy has an advantage, since without the complete devotion of both parents, the male and the female, the species and its genes might not be able to survive.

Future studies may one day reveal that the way in which such a change occurs in nature in response to environmental conditions is through epigenetics. Epigenetic paternity is passed down through the sperm cells from father to son, as we saw in the study of the mice that passed the fear of the smell of vanilla to their offspring in one generation following a change in their environmental conditions.

Since that 2016 study, researchers in Dr Larry Young's lab have also deciphered the neural pathways that enable monogamy; that is, the specific neural pathways in the pleasure and reward system in the brains of monogamous prairie voles, which are responsible for their falling in love and becoming attached. The researchers examined the brains of the voles after their first sexual contact, to see how falling in love affects their brains in terms of their neural pathways. Falling in love is linked to the same neural pathways that connect the image and smell of the beloved to reward and pleasure. Moreover, the researchers were even able to make a virgin vole fall in love through a glass window with another virgin, without physical contact taking place and without orgasm occurring. They were able to produce the infatuation through artificial external stimulation of the same neural pathways of oxytocin in the pleasure system of the female's brain. The stimulation was achieved using optogenetic technology, which enables the turning on or off of individual neurons or a pathway in the brain using genetic engineering and fibre optics.

In the future, will it be possible to go to brain therapy instead of marriage counselling and create a wonderful lifelong loving relationship, just by periodically stimulating electrodes within the pleasure and reward system of our brain?

Monogamy and Parenting

One of the most prominent characteristics of monogamous versus polygamous animals concerns parental behaviour and the equal sharing of the burden of parenting between the male and the female, or joint parenting. This is in contrast to polygamous animals, in which parenting is the exclusive task of the female. The question arises as to whether the parental skills of monogamous males and females are heredity or environmentally influenced. Are the skills passed only in the genes or caused by the surroundings as well? This is exactly the question that interested Dr Hopi Hoekstra at Harvard in 2017, when she delved into the genetics of monogamy and parental behaviour. Hoekstra wondered what would happen if she took a male born to polygamous parents and let monogamous parents raise him from the day he was born: would he grow up to be monogamous like his adoptive father, or polygamous like his biological father?

To examine the question, Hoekstra took the mouse pups of polygamous parents and gave them to rare monogamous oldfield mice parents to raise them. Although the offspring of polygamous parents were raised by devoted monogamous fathers, their genetics prevailed. The sons of polygamous fathers exhibited exactly the same polygamous behaviour as their biological fathers and didn't care for their own offspring at all, even though they grew up with monogamous fathers. Their dedicated and caring monogamous father figure didn't affect their own behaviour as such.

In the second step, to decipher the regions of the genome responsible for the monogamous parental behaviour in the oldfield mice, Hoekstra mated five polygamous mice and five monogamous oldfield mice. Their offspring were also mated with each other, resulting in 770 hybrid offspring. The genome of these 770 hybrid offspring is essentially a mosaic of their monogamous and polygamous parents. In the next step, Hoekstra observed the behaviour of the 770 offspring. Surprisingly, she saw a wide range of parental behaviours: there were those who did not take care of the offspring at all, some who took care of them in a slightly slapdash manner but did not build impressive nests, while others behaved just like the monogamous oldfield mice and some even became devoted parents who licked their offspring constantly and spent a lot of time building luxurious nests.

The range of the males' behaviours, from extreme polygamous behaviour to extreme monogamy, allowed the researchers to examine and compare DNA sequences and the specific genes that are responsible for each behaviour and are expressed differently in the various mice. They found, for example, a certain region of the genome that greatly influences nest building. There was usually not one segment but a variety of segments that influenced several behaviours, such as one region of the genome that was responsible for the following four traits: how long parents lick their pups, how much they cuddle up with them, how long they stay with them, and how quickly they reunited with the pups after the researchers temporarily remove them from the nest. Hoekstra and her team found that there were sequences of the genome more important for male parental behaviour than for female parental behaviour, and vice versa. This suggests that males and females diverged on different evolutionary paths toward monogamous parenting and toward monogamy in general. This divergence also manifests itself in the development of the male version of the hormone oxytocin, vasopressin, which produces different parental and marital behaviour.

Are Humans Naturally Monogamous or Polygamous?

The study of monogamy at the level of genetics, neurology and biochemistry is still in its infancy. Many more discoveries are expected that will shed light on the biological basis of monogamy in humans as well as in other animals. These discoveries, it can be assumed, will change how we look at the way we bond and the variety of factors that influence our relationship behaviours, some of which we didn't really know existed until about two decades ago. It is possible that one day, when the genetics of love have been completely deciphered, and each of us can hold our genome in the palm of our hand, as a file on our mobile, dating apps will automatically offer us matches based on our personal DNA.

Do we humans belong to the polygamous group, like 97 per cent of mammals, or do we actually belong to the monogamous group, like some birds and a rare 3 per cent of mammals? This is an unsolved question that scientists grapple with, and there are arguments for and against both sides of the equation. With humans, everything is more complex and depends on many socio-cultural factors that differ from one society to another, and which may change over time.

On the one hand, if we look at the mammals closest to us genetically on the evolutionary tree, the apes, gorillas, chimpanzees, the bonobo and the orangutan, they all seem to lead a polygamous lifestyle. All but the gibbons. Gibbons are a species of short-nosed primates that are at home in the tropical forests of Southeast Asia. Unlike other apes, gibbons live a monogamous lifestyle and maintain a nuclear family, usually consisting of a couple and an infant. The baby gibbon stays with the parents until it's about eight years old, when it becomes independent. And what happens when the gibbon leaves? Do his parents stay together for life? The gibbons probably belong to the serial monogamous group, as they sometimes change partners when the child leaves and also cheat on each other during their life together.

To answer the question of which group we belong to, whether the polygamous or the monogamous (and let's be realistic – considering the frequency of betrayal and divorce among humans, we're at best "serial-monogamous"), we will examine the arguments for and against.

First, let's examine how monogamous males differ from polygamous males. The monogamous males are very similar to the females. Since they are essential for the care of the offspring and don't need to impress all the females all the time and fight with other males, they don't have unnecessary adornments like feathers, horns or war paint. They look almost like the female and their testosterone levels are relatively low compared to that of the polygamous males; in fact, it's similar to the levels found in females.

In comparison, the polygamous males are often larger than the females in terms of their body mass and muscles, and may be decorated with horns, feathers, impressive colours and more. All these outward signs are a product of their high testosterone at work, and are secondary sex markings, which begin to appear at puberty and intensify as the polygamous male wins more battles and enjoys success with the females.

And as for us humans? Although our males do not have feathers, horns or warning colours, their testosterone levels are 15 to 100 times higher than female levels. This explains why men are larger than women in body mass by 15 per cent on average, and their muscle mass to fat ratio is higher compared to that of women. Men have muscle under the skin while women have subcutaneous fat and under that is the muscle. Men's body structure and facial structure are different; they are more hirsute and their voices are deeper. All these male secondary sex signs look very attractive to women.

And what about a man's penis and testicles? The level of testosterone also affects the testicles and the penis, which is why in monogamous species the penis and the testicles are relatively small, and we mentioned earlier how the vast majority of bird species have lost their penis completely. We also mentioned that the prize for the largest penis and testicles relative to body mass in the entire animal kingdom . . . goes to men. The penis and testicles of the human are proportionally the largest in the entire animal kingdom.

(As a side note, the size of the testicles is related to the amount of sperm they produce, as demonstrated in 2011 by a group of great ape researchers from Tokai University in Japan. The researchers compared the testicular tissues of chimpanzees, orangutans and gorillas and found huge variations. They discovered that the sperm-producing tissues in the gorilla's testicles were thinner than those of the orangutan and chimpanzee. They also found that chimpanzees produce 14 times more sperm than orangutans and 200 times more than gorillas. In other words, the Japanese scientists were able to prove that the size of the testicles is indeed related to sperm production.)

On average, the human testicles weigh about twenty grams each and are big in relation to our body size. They are more similar (in terms of their size relative to the body) to chimpanzee and bonobo testicles than to gorilla and gibbon testicles, suggesting some level of sperm competition in humans. That is, men need to produce a lot of sperm because they have many competitors for the hearts and bodies of women. As we have seen, 80 per cent of sperm cells are used to attack and inhibit other men's sperm.

More significant scientific proof of the competitiveness of sperm in humans was found in a genetic study carried out at the University of Chicago in the United States in 2003. The researchers analysed the sequence of two genes (SEMG1 and SEMG2), which encode certain proteins found in seminal fluid. The role of these proteins is to cause the sperm to coagulate immediately after ejaculation, when it is inside the vagina and cervix, and to create lumps of sperm called "mating plugs". As mentioned briefly in chapter 7, the purpose of a mating plug is to prevent new sperm from competitors from entering the female's vagina. These sperm protein-specific genes are only found in the genomes of males of animals that have high sperm competition; in other words, when females have several partners with whom they mate and there is a lot of competition between the males. The researchers identified a direct relationship between the average number of sexual partners females have in different species, and the presence of these genes for sperm proteins in the males' genome; they found that the more partners females have on average, the more these genes appear. The findings of the studies seem to suggest that monogamy has not been the central strategy of the human species throughout evolution.

As we have already seen, in humans there is a great difference in appearance between men and women, men have proportionally large testicles and there is the presence of genes for sperm proteins that suggest sperm competition. We also have to take into consideration the Coolidge effect, which causes the level of sexual excitement to decrease after spending some time with the same partner. All of this differs from standard monogamous traits. In addition, men create a rigid hierarchy and fight each other just like the polygamist species do. In virtually every social structure of ours, there exists a hierarchy, and this often has the same hierarchical pattern as that of polygamists: a dominance hierarchy. In a dominance hierarchy, each individual tries to control other individuals and everyone is collectively subordinate to the alpha male. We find such hierarchies in the family unit, in the military, in the workplace and in the political arena. There is always one leader, one head of the family, a chief of staff, director general, general secretary, prime minister, president or king. Masculine characteristics, high in testosterone, have always been linked to leadership: an imposing physical presence, a height advantage, charisma, a willingness to take risks and a coldness of spirit. Our entire history is about alpha males, their wars and struggles for control – kings, emperors and generals, all high on testosterone, low in empathy, and driven by ego and power. As a general principle, only men go to war on conquest and killing campaigns, annexing new territories and accumulating land as a reward for victory in battle.

In times of war, the men kill the cubs (children), commit genocide and rape girls and women, destroying competing genes with violent and cruel seed distribution. In terms of human evolution, these methods have been successful; the ultimate alpha male of the human species, the man whose genes are most widely scattered in the population, is none other than the psychopathic paedophile and brutal murderer Genghis Khan. Genghis Khan lived around 850 years ago, and according to a major study, one in five Asian men carries his genes on the Y chromosome. This extrapolates to 1 in every 200 men in the world. We cannot deny the fact that most of us are the descendants of men's conquests and wars.

For humans, power, control and reproduction have always gone hand in hand, similar to other polygamous species. Privileges of reproduction belong to the ruling male, and kings or emperors have traditionally always had the greatest number of descendants across different cultures. The Inca Empire in South America, for example, had a highly controlled breeding industry.

The Inca law book did not deal with government and public policy, but with how many wives a man was allowed to marry according to his position in the social hierarchy: the king was allowed to marry 1,500 wives, nobles could have 700 wives, governors 50, and so on, down to men of the lowest rank, the poor, who according to the law were allowed just one. Polygamy was decreed for the rich and monogamy reserved only for the poor.

We can look around today and see that, while rare, polygamy still exists among humans. It remains a way of life among some Arab peoples and in sub-Saharan Africa, for example. The concept of romantic love is relatively new and exists mainly in the Western world. In biblical times, for example, polygamy was a common way of life and the ancient Israelites married several wives. This way of life continued until Rabbi Gershom regulated against polygamy, overturning rules that were followed within the Jewish diaspora in Europe around a thousand years ago.

Before Rabbi Gershom's ban on polygamy, a man was allowed to have multiple wives, as long as he was able to give them all food, clothing and sexual relations. When Rabbi Gershom instituted his ban, he cited several reasons for encouraging monogamy. He sought to prevent the domineering and violent behaviour of men toward their wives, especially acts of theft and debauchery, and to promote peace and calm, because multiple wives can lead to jealousy and quarrels. And Rabbi Gershom also considered the household budget, as with each additional woman a new family is potentially created, and in a situation that is under financial stress that could be a recipe for disaster.

In a survey of 1,231 cultures, conducted between 1960 and 1980, the American anthropologist George Murdoch found 588 groups with a high incidence of polygamy, 453 groups with a small percentage of polygamy, four groups engaged in polyandry (in which a woman has several male partners) and 186 monogamous cultures. In most cases where polygamy is allowed, the number of men who have more than one wife is limited, because of the need for a level of material resources not available to everyone. In some societies, multiple wives are a status symbol for a man. Even in monogamous societies, having a kept woman or mistress in addition to a legal wife, or having multiple partners, can be a way to indicate a high status for the men.

Studies have found that polygamy remains more common in disease-prone areas, especially in tropical zones, leading to the hypothesis that in such places the genes promoting polygamy tend to survive better because of the very high infant mortality rate.

Our environment definitely affects reproduction and lifestyle, and pushes societies to favour one or the other reproductive strategy. In Tibet, for example, there is a severe shortage of agricultural land in the Himalayas. Here, the rare strategy of polyandry takes hold, where a woman will marry several men, usually brothers. In these instances, the appeal of polyandry is that it prevents the fragmentation of the few available agricultural areas into small plots, which would not be enough to support a family. Another factor that leads to the existence of polyandry in certain Asian societies is the cruel practice of killing female infants, which reduces the number of women in the population. In contrast to the extremes of female infanticide, in certain tribes along the banks of the Amazon, women believe that in order to give birth to a smart, strong, tall and funny child, you would need to sleep with the smart guy, the strong guy, the tall guy and the funny guy of the tribe so that all their sperm will mix and bestow these features on your child.

A Short History of Monogamy

Monogamy, as we have seen, is a relatively new concept for *Homo sapiens*. The main argument of those who believe that man is biologically monogamous is that our offspring are born helpless. A human baby remains helpless for the longest time in the animal kingdom and needs a lot of long-term care. A child also demands huge resources and may sometimes even stay in the parental home until the age of thirty. Therefore, two parents are needed to take care of the offspring until they grow up and can raise offspring themselves.

Monogamy in human societies is practised in Europe, Eurasia and America and is related to socio-cultural processes. The Romans first spread the practice via the influence of Christianity in their colonies across Europe and Asia. However, this had nothing to do with true love and everything to do with the need to control men in their territories in such a way that they would not rebel. In a polygamous system, the clan is often a powerful unit, acting like small armies in which the men are primarily loyal to the clan and its chieftain and thereby making it difficult to establish a central government in the area. (To this day, polygamy and clan structures make governance and the establishment of central rule difficult in certain Arab and African countries.) The Romans decided to break the clan mechanism by preventing polygamy and encouraging monogamy instead. The theory went that if you could imprison a man in the institution of marriage with one wife and the equivalent of a mortgage and three children, he would no longer rebel against the Empire and would be much more obedient. The method was successful and the Empire won. This is how monogamy slowly took hold of the human race and enabled progress and development. The idea of monogamous romantic love took root throughout the Christian world through the influence of social institutions and later through the agents of literature, theatre, cinema, television and in every possible new form of media.

As we have seen, humans are very complex creatures and our behaviour depends on so many different environmental factors – whether biological, social or cultural – and our form of monogamy is undoubtedly social-serial. From around the 1970s, divorce became much easier in the West and the feminist revolution led to a surge in women's rights, including the ability to get custody of the children and support them herself. The model of lifelong monogamy, "till death do us part", collapsed like a house of cards. The institution of marriage remains in decline, while the divorce rate continues to increase, and the average time between getting married and divorce among young people today is somewhere between two and three years. Today human behaviour lies somewhere between serial monogamy and polyamory – multiple partners – and all this has happened within a few generations.

My Israeli grandmother, for example, married at the beginning of the last century at the age of 20 to a man 20 years her senior and had no choice in the matter. In the 1970s, my mother married her sweetheart but stayed at home to raise the children and was completely dependent on her husband. Whereas today, at the age of 44, I had already managed to divorce twice, raised two wonderful children as a single parent and entered into relationships entirely of my own choosing. And all this has happened in the span of only three generations . . .

CHAPTER 9
THE FUTURE OF LOVE

What does the future look like for human relationships? To find some answers, perhaps we could begin by checking our genome. Do we carry the "monogamy gene" like prairie voles do, or do we carry the polygamy version like meadow voles? What do genetics tell us about our love patterns?

These questions interested Dr Hasse Walum from the Karolinska Institute in Sweden in 2008. Walum wanted to find out if the human male genome has the same genetic alteration that causes the prairie voles to be monogamous. For this purpose, Walum and his team examined the genetic data of 600 Swedish men who were either identical or non-identical twins, and living in a relationship. In the next step, they asked the partners of the male twins to rate their degree of monogamy with questions such as: *How much affection does your partner show you? How good do you think he is in the relationship? How faithful is he? How much does he participate in raising the children?* And so on.

The researchers then checked the male twins' genome sequence for the "monogamy gene". They specifically looked at the same gene for the vasopressin receptor, the male version of oxytocin or the love hormone, which differed in the monogamous prairie voles compared to their polygamous cousins. This gene, like many genes of the emotional mechanisms, is highly conserved throughout evolution, so it is possible to compare the form of the gene in men with the form found in prairie voles. The findings showed that there is a difference in the sequence of the "monogamy gene" between different men, and that the male twins whose gene form was more similar to that of the prairie voles were also rated as more monogamous by their female partners.

In addition, the researchers noticed a significant difference in the configuration of the "monogamy gene" between different men, with the gene undergoing various kinds of changes. In the wake of that study in Sweden, an American genetics company that supplies genetic sequencing for $120 now offers a genetic test for monogamy in men. Anyone wishing to check the degree of their partner's monogamy can simply collect a DNA sample from saliva or other bodily fluids and have it analysed in a laboratory.

So do genetics finally solve the riddle of who we are? Walum's research shows that in humans, too, the genes associated with monogamy play a role and influence our degree of satisfaction in a single, long-term relationship, and the level of sexual excitement that we continue to find with the same partner. The genetics of love is a fascinating field in which many more discoveries are expected, such as deciphering the genes relating to relationship and parental behaviour, as well as the various ways in which our environment affects our biology and genetics – the epigenetics of relationship behaviours. At this stage, we are still far from fully understanding the set of genetic, biological, environmental and cultural factors that influence our love lives and our choices over time. No man is exactly the same as his friend, nor is any woman just like her sister; we are all a mosaic of biological, psychological and cultural components that influence our behaviour in relationships.

We probably never belonged to the group of sexually monogamous species who stay together for life – and never will. Humans move on a continuum between serial monogamy and polygamy or polyamory, depending on their circumstances. We are very sexual creatures, the most sexual in the living world, and also very flexible in our sexuality, which can make us more confused than ever today about who we really are, what suits us and what society demands or should even demand of us. As far as our genes are concerned, they will probably continue to push us not to put all our eggs in one basket, but to spread the risk by having multiple partners, especially those with good genes.

All this is subject to the options available in our environment. The ecology of love decrees that it is our surroundings that dictate the sexual behaviours of all species on Earth. In an environment of scarcity – when there are not enough resources, the threats are many and both parents are needed for the survival of the offspring – the genetic selection will be in favour of monogamy. However, in an environment of abundance, when there is a surplus of resources and the investment of one parent is enough for the offspring to survive and thrive, our genes will favour multiple partners and greater competition.

Since the environment inhabited by humans has also changed significantly over the generations, from scarcity to abundance, of both resources and the availability of temptations, there may be ever more difficulties in maintaining monogamy. The modern age of plenty is especially challenging for monogamy; it is not for nothing that some call it "the age of the singleton" – an era characterized by the rising numbers of single mothers who choose to have a child with donated sperm. Where I live, in Israel, there was a 30 per cent increase in the decade from 2005 to 2015. Reports from England in 2023 indicate more children were born from sperm donation than from the old-fashioned method.

When we consider sperm donation, this suggests a return to a certain type of polygamy. No woman walks into a sperm bank and asks to pick a random sample out of the cooler. She meticulously leafs through a catalogue showing the genetic assets of various men. She makes a sexual selection from the catalogue, choosing the best genes in her eyes. She will usually choose educated, highly intelligent, muscular men with chiselled features, or in other words, as close to an alpha as possible. There are many young, handsome and anonymous doctors whose genes are scattered throughout the population.

As a counter-movement to cold and mechanical sperm banks, an independent sperm movement has arisen; men can offer their sperm for free, anonymously. One such site is the Known Donor Registry, which has 13,000 registrations. Profiles used on the site range from "get good genes into your womb" to "let me make you a mother". There are donors in their 30s and 40s who have already donated their sperm to dozens of women. They describe the excitement they feel when a woman announces that she has had a positive pregnancy test and another child of theirs is about to emerge into the world.

Indeed, even in 2023, as at the dawn of history on Earth, genes are the ones running the show. The story of Dr Jan Karbaat, manager of a sperm bank in the Netherlands, who fathered children with his own sperm, stands out. At least 60 children were apparently created from his sperm, without the consent and knowledge of the women, and the scam was only discovered when parents began to notice over the years that their children resembled the doctor who managed the sperm bank.

Although the females of animals belonging to polygamous species do not technically have the option of fertilizing themselves with donated sperm, the selection process they carry out is essentially no different from the process that humans use. They acquire a male's genes without any real need for his physical investment in their offspring. What will happen when the technology that already exists today is used to fertilize an egg from the DNA of another egg or from any other cell, without a particular need for sperm? What will be the fate of men then? The American journalist Hanna Rosin wrestles with these questions in her book *The End of Men: And the Rise of Women*, in which she posits that we find ourselves in a historical moment where the changes experienced by women in recent decades mean they are speeding forward while leaving men behind in the dust. But where does this leave us now?

What Does the Future Hold for Loving Relationships?

"We are probably not a classical pairwise monogamous species, nor a classical competitive polygamous species. What we are, officially, is a tragically confused species," wrote renowned researcher Professor Robert Sapolsky. In this confused age of ours, on the one hand, we are disillusioned with Disney-style romances about princesses waiting for handsome princes with whom they will live happily ever after. And, on the other hand, we yearn for strong and stable relationships; we want to form a lasting bond with one person, someone who will really get to know us and love us and we will love that person in return.

Today, many of us are trying to reimagine what our relationships might look like and we are turning to biology for help. There are those voices that tell us: *Why oppose our natural instincts? We are not naturally monogamous. All this monogamy is a conspiracy of empires new and old, and their elites. We should not be the victims of society. Let's free ourselves from our shackles: it's in our nature to love freely, so why limit ourselves to sex and love with one person for life?* Within this discourse, a number of models exist for coping with the challenges of monogamy and especially for dealing with the Coolidge effect, the reality of excitement fading over time.

One model is that of the open relationship, in which a couple consensually experiences casual sexual encounters outside of the traditional romantic-marital-family context. However, the couple usually don't share the details of their sexual exploits with each other in order not to arouse jealousy or to spoil the long-term relationship. This is an intermediate type of monogamy with wandering eyes, which has been called "monogamish".

Couples reach an open relationship model for a variety of reasons. Perhaps the couple is a little bored with sex, feel overly familiar with each other's bodies and want to regain the thrill of tremendous orgasms. The couple acknowledges any differences in each other's sex drive; for example, perhaps one of them needs sex more often, while the other is more focused on friendship, security and the emotional side of the relationship.

However, whether it's down to biology or the social conventions that are ingrained in us, most couples don't manage to maintain open relationships for long. Sometimes couples pay the price when uncontrollable jealousy arises; if, say, one of them finds it difficult to bear even just the thought of what their partner does with someone else, while they themselves are not particularly interested in pursuing adventures with new sexual partners.

It is often necessary to engage in therapy as a couple in order to have an open relationship and for it to stay healthy. This is because in terms of biology, the love hormone we know as oxytocin does not distinguish sexual encounters from love. When we have sex with others we can readily fall in love with them; the same chemistry works in the brain even if we ourselves define the relationship as temporary. New thrills will always be stronger than the old and familiar, so a decrease in intercourse and intimate contact with the permanent partner ensues, causing a decline in oxytocin and increased distancing, certainly when accompanied by acute feelings of jealousy and frustration. However, in some cases, the fact that the partner is sexually desired by others can cause an increase in sexual excitement, and the couple's own sex life actually improves and the relationship strengthens between them.

Alongside the debate on flexible monogamy that allows for the occasional sexual flings of both partners, there is also a growing discussion about polyamory, and the polyamorous community is growing globally. Polyamory is a lifestyle that includes having love-based relationships with more than one partner, with the consent of all parties. Polyamorous situations are often hierarchical, in which the relationship consists of a central partner and several secondary lovers. With the main partner, it's usual to manage a joint household, raise children and eat meals as a family unit. On a parallel track, each partner has secondary lovers. There is no orderly and clear difference. Just as monogamous couples have a unique discourse about their relationship and intimacy, so too do polyamorous couples formulate and jointly examine what is good for them and where their boundaries lie.

In polyamorous relationships, it's natural that jealousy should pose a more complex challenge since we are not talking about a passing sexual encounter with another individual, but a real love relationship. However, it is not always easy to come to terms with the fact that your partner loves not only you but also other people, and they provide your partner with other emotional needs besides sex. Jealousy may be a product of biology or of the culture we live in, or both; whichever it is, there is no doubt that it is present and can provoke many conflicts within a polyamorous system.

For this reason, anyone entering into polyamory must be long-suffering and have an enormous amount of patience. People who have chosen polyamory admit that jealousy is indeed a dominant emotion, but that they deal with it in a different way. According to them, it isn't destructive but a healthy form of jealousy that is not driven by possessiveness. The polyamorous lifestyle stems from a great love for a partner and a desire to make him or her happy, even if this is at the expense of the partner who gives up exclusivity. According to the polyamorous, we were taught a certain way of life and now they are trying something different, which requires open-mindedness and a change of habits. Polyamory requires much more time and energy than monogamy, because it involves maintaining several relationships, and in our frenzied world it often seems difficult to find time even for one of them. Investing in several relationships means less shared time with the main partner, less oxytocin in connection to them and a relationship that may weaken and be damaged by a lack of attention. Quite a few monogamous relationships are wrecked by a distancing and diminishing investment in the relationship.

There are also some professionals, such as philosophy professor Carrie Jenkins from Columbia University in the United States, who enthusiastically support the polyamorous lifestyle. In her book *What Love Is: And What It Could Be*, Jenkins asserts that society's perception of romantic love is too narrow and exclusive. Just because the social order does not include polyamory, this does not mean that it is not legitimate; on the contrary, it is a reason to challenge the social structure with additional possibilities. According to her, romantic love can be divided into a biological component and a social component. Biologically, our brain chemistry for love doesn't require monogamy, or one relationship with one person. But society today defines romantic love only in its monogamous form and anything else is deemed to be improper. In her view, the same sort of coercion exists regarding the model of heterosexuality, but we must not coerce people into making a choice that does not suit them. When we decide there is only one way suitable for everyone, we force people to live inside a single box, a life that is not healthy for them.

This statement is also fully supported by biology. Genetic studies show that we are very different from each other in everything related to the mechanics of love and other emotional processes. What suits one person will not necessarily suit another. Since we are an intermediate generation, finding ourselves in a transitional phase between an old world where there is only one way to live and a new world where all lifestyles are acceptable, we are very confused. The conventions, norms and hidden messages of society and our parents still live on in our minds and in the minds of our spouses, so when we try to make changes in order to be happier, it can be important to seek professional help so as not to fall into distressing and destructive relationship conflicts.

CHAPTER 10

THE PRESCRIPTION FOR LONG-LASTING LOVE

We are definitely a complicated generation. With our own hands, we have smashed the mechanisms of a social order that lasted, in one form or another, for tens of thousands of years. These structures preserved the balance of power in society and were based on hierarchy, control and dependence.

Women and children were once owned by the man at the head of the family, and everyone was clear about their place in the family structure. Indeed, the very word "family" originates from the Latin *famulus*, meaning servant. The social norms related to the structure of the family and the power positions of men and women in relation to each other were passed down from generation to generation, from mother to daughter and father to son, and in this way the social order was preserved.

The roots of these social structures can be found in our biology and exist in other animals. The urge to control and prove paternity is older than humankind, and it no longer suits us. We want to transcend biology. We are neither animals nor chimpanzees. Nor are we puppets with DNA pulling our strings. We don't want to be held captive by our genes. We wish to build new structures, a new social order. The institution of marriage is out, the era of the supreme male is over. We want to create an equal marital system, without struggles for power and control, free from gender expectations and free from the intervention of the state. Today, we are not prepared to sacrifice ourselves in a relationship or to give up what we can have.

But to add to our confusion, we still haven't acquired the tools that will allow us to live in an equal relationship; we had nowhere to buy them. We are the first generation that dares to rebel, and the establishment is certainly not helping us. The social political structures have not changed at the rate we have evolved, and they have no interest in changing. The world of work is mostly still built on a gender division of roles, visible or hidden, where men are expected to work long hours and be 100 per cent focused on their tasks in order to climb the organizational ladder. And from their point of view, the care of the children is the responsibility of the woman. The number of women who step off the career ladder after having children remains large. Many women also leave prized positions because the male work environment and organizational culture are not geared toward their needs.

A fundamental historical social injustice, and a major obstacle to creating an equal relationship, is that the work of caring for children at home is unpaid labour and not included in national accounting (GDP) and the economy. Even in 2021, studies show how in Western countries women still do 70 per cent of the work in raising children and taking care of the home. When discussing his famous question, "How do you get your dinner?", Adam Smith, the father of capitalism, pointed to the baker who sells the bread, the brewer who makes the beer and the butcher who sells the meat, and explained that everyone does this for their own benefit and not for ours. But who did Smith forget? Who cooked, prepared and served his own dinner? Whose Sisyphean hard work did Smith neglect to include in his economic analysis? His mother's. Smith was a bachelor who lived with his devoted mother, who cared for him, served his meals and took care of the housework so that her talented son could quietly immerse himself in his studies.

Women contribute countless hours of free labour – input which does not appear in the national accounting, even though the economy relies on it. This reliance is both at the level of making routine economic activity possible and in the important job of raising future productive citizens. The women are often the unseen labourers and their work is invisible.

Moreover, when women become mothers they often experience systematic discrimination in the workplace – discrimination in pay, hiring, benefits, promotion and an unfavourable perception of their abilities compared to women without children. Mothers are seen as less committed to their paid jobs, less responsible and also less authoritative than women without children. This phenomenon has been called the "motherhood penalty". Today, divorced fathers sharing joint custody of their children can also suffer from a "paternity penalty", but women still remain more affected and suffer a double penalty for each additional child. One can only assume that the world of work and the economy would look completely different if the task of creating life and nurturing it was performed by men.

The underestimation of women or anything perceived as feminine is also seen in the wage gap between the sexes. Women's salaries are, on average, 30 per cent lower than men's, and average pay in professions considered "female" – the "oxytocin professions" of teaching, caring and nursing – is half of what people expect to earn in professions considered masculine, the more technological "testosterone professions". This reality creates a great economic dependence of women on men, which dictates the power relations in society. Today, 95 per cent of global capital is still concentrated in the hands of men.

In light of this reality, it is no wonder that we encounter so many difficulties when we try to create an equal relationship. As long as the social structures remain unequal, many couples experience recurring crises, mainly around child-raising and the tensions between career and family. The conflict stems from the desires of both spouses for fulfilment and self-realization while building and nurturing a family. And if we add in the Coolidge effect, we face some serious challenges in sustaining a committed loving relationship "till death do us part".

If we look at the list of the most common conflicts between spouses, the ones that usually come up in marriage counselling, the top-ranked conflict is over the division of labour. In second place are disputes around sex, which will usually be a by-product of other disputes combined with the Coolidge effect. Third place goes to disputes around the education and care of children. In the fourth place are disputes over money. And in the fifth place, we hear about conflicts over relations with the in-laws.

Added to this list are issues related to jealousy: arguments about not showing enough affection and attention, outbursts of anger, power struggles, poor communication or thunderous silences, disputes over leisure time, lack of appreciation, the feeling that one partner is trying to change the other, and problems of trust.

Ninety per cent of fights between spouses are recurring arguments about the same grudge with minor variations. Sixty-five per cent of these rows have no solution. They are simply a means of releasing accumulated pressures and tensions. The same conflicts keep recurring because these fixed patterns of behaviour can be difficult to change, and the normal form of communication between the couple doesn't resolve them. The reason these issues stir up turbulent emotions, escalating into emotional quarrels, is that they relate to the basic needs of one or both of the spouses, which are not being met. As previously noted, an emotion we feel implies a need. Emotion is a gift, and whatever evokes strong emotions in us implies that it touches our essential needs, which are sometimes difficult for us to convey to another party.

Looking at long-term loving relationships in a rational and scientific way, through the prefrontal cortex and not through the emotional brain, allows us to detach ourselves for a moment from the deep emotional involvement in the issue and get a bird's-eye view from which to examine the difficulties, barriers and crises that all couples experience at some point in their relationship. So what leads some couples to overcome their difficulties and others to break up? What are the pitfalls that can be expected and how can we avoid falling into traps we know about in advance? From this wider perspective, we can create tools based on our understanding of the brain, biology and science, and apply them to ourselves when we come to build a happy and healthy, long-term relationship. This is assuming we want one, of course . . .

Humans have the freedom to choose and a mind with which to explore options. We can choose what is good for us. No woman is alike, and no two men are the same. We come in a tremendous variety of types and wiring. Only we know what is good for us and when. Only we know in which types of relationships we flourish and when we wither. Looking directly at who we really are, at what is good for us and also at what is not good for us, allows us to free ourselves from the shackles that hold us back. And, of course, we also change during the course of life. Our brain develops and adapts over time, we see things differently at different ages and our needs themselves change. What was good for us at 20 does not necessarily suit us at 30, 40 or 60. We gain life experience, new synapses are formed in our brains, and our thinking changes.

Women change, men change, social structures change, and we live in an age of free choice. There is no right and wrong, no forbidden and permitted, and this brings freedom and liberation but also great confusion. This is called the paradox of multiple choice. Precisely when all the options are in front of us, it's difficult to reach a decision. We hate the idea of losing, we fear missing out and are prone to many more biases. Sometimes it's actually convenient for us to have people decide for us, as then all we have to do is complain.

Monogamy may be maligned, but studies show that people who live in a good monogamous relationship are generally healthier, happier and live longer (thanks to the oxytocin). Monogamy offers certainty, security, mental support, emotional stability and the ability to bond deeply with one person. The journey of life includes ups and downs, moments of pain and moments of happiness; it is a great privilege to share those moments with a loyal travelling companion. Recent happiness studies show that the best thing a heterosexual man can do for his happiness is to marry a woman, and for a woman it's to expand her circle of friends. The obvious conclusion is that the company of women boosts oxytocin.

Now that we know what love is biologically, and we also understand the cultural roots of monogamy as we know it today – and from our own free choice, with no strings attached, we choose stable and safe monogamous love, for all its advantages and disadvantages – it's time to equip ourselves with a research-based toolbox that will help us to enjoy a successful journey. I call it "Dr Liat Yakir's scientific prescription for preserving conjugal love":

Let's Learn to Choose Correctly

One of the most important choices we can make in life, which has the strongest effect on our happiness, is the choice of the partner with whom we hope to raise a family. We can switch careers, find a new workplace or move house as we see fit, but we cannot change the mother or father of our children, so this choice stays with us throughout our lives. However, since the emotional brain manages this selection process, and it works seven times faster than the rational brain, it is difficult for us to exercise full discretion in choosing our spouses. In addition, when we are under the influence of the chemicals of love, during the time of falling in love, the ability to make decisions goes completely haywire and we sometimes get carried away by choices that are not necessarily good for us.

However, now that we understand how our brain works when it comes to love, and how difficult it is for us to exercise judgement and see reality for what it truly is when we are in love, perhaps this new awareness can help us manage the process, instead of the process managing us.

They say that to understand something means to be free of it. Awareness makes up half of this. During a new relationship, it's important to check for warning signs. Take note of whether your intended has traits or behaviour patterns you find challenging to deal with. Try to make sure you are not repeating patterns from the past. Ask yourself how motivated you are by fear or stress. If doubts arise, you should talk to the people who love you and want your best; they might see things more clearly, since their minds are not flooded with love chemicals.

But do be careful of rumination – that tendency to deal with things in a repetitive and circular manner, which hinders rather than helps. If you feel you are repeating inhibiting relationship patterns, or experience difficulty in forming a bond with someone, especially if you have known trauma in the past, please help your brain heal from past experiences and cut off the negative conditioning before you go looking for a relationship. Your choices and your loves will look completely different once your mind is freed from the distressing factors it clings to from the past.

While practising this sort of rational thinking, it is always important to remember the mathematics of love in the selection process. Although the emotional mind refuses to believe it, let's remember that the probability of finding the "one" or the one that ticks all our boxes is 1 in 562, which is ten times more difficult than our chances of becoming a millionaire. There really isn't that one perfect partner out there who is smart, funny, handsome, grounded, ambitious, a perfect lover, an exemplary parent, kind, sensitive and interested in the same things as you; those are ten different people. A better course of action is to choose according to the features that are more relevant to creating a family unit, establishing a solid base and building a relationship for the long term. These qualities are different from those that are important in a tumultuous and short-lived sensual affair. In many cases, we may not feel butterflies in the stomach, a pounding heart and a stirring in the genitals on our first date. These physiological phenomena are a product of oxytocin, the love hormone, and it takes time to produce oxytocin with a person we've just met. It requires proximity, quality time and shared experiences, intimacy, mutual support, trust building and then, like a magic wand, oxytocin floods the bloodstream, awakens those butterflies in the stomach, raises your blood pressure and creates the same euphoric feeling that suddenly causes the potential candidate to appear more beautiful, more attractive and stimulating. The tragedy is that we often don't give oxytocin a chance.

The multitude of options out there drives us crazy, and we quickly rule some out and swipe left to consider the next one. It's important to remember that without oxytocin, the magic that is love will not happen. This is why the digital world is so damaging to people's ability to bond with others; it decreases the level of oxytocin while at the same time producing the white noise of stimuli. That's why it's important to be smart in the online dating arena and keep your head. Let's remember that the business model of the tech sector is not built on the success of a long-term relationship but on the time the user spends in the app. I would also like to remind you that a dating app is actually a Skinner box (see page 35), which drives the brain's dopamine reward system crazy. Over time, numbness sets in and the negativity bias increases, which manifests itself in over-filtering, harsh judgement and criticism that intensify after each disappointing date or ghosting (disappearance). Therefore, make sure to limit your time in dating apps, take a break from time to time, spend more time with friends and take more initiative to meet people offline. We know that there is no substitute for eye contact, nor is there a substitute for natural oxytocin.

Another insight worth remembering from the field of love mathematics, regarding when to stop searching, is the solution to the problem of optimization. After going out with 37 per cent of the potential candidates we could meet during our lifetime, it is worth settling down with the first one we meet after age 28 (or 30 for men) who is better than all the predecessors. There's no point in dragging this decision out too long, the possibilities are endless, and 30 is not the new 20, at least not in terms of the biological clock in the womb. Age 28 to 30 is a good time because this is when the prefrontal cortex completes its development, and our rational thinking finally takes shape. As mentioned, in women the prefrontal cortex develops about two to four years faster than in men. Therefore, the feeling that women sometimes have about men – that they are a little late to mature – is based to some extent on brain research.

It is also worth remembering that we are often drawn to the different, but studies show that in the end, we stick with the familiar. We may be attracted to people who are different from us in character or come from a different culture – genes look for genetic diversity – but studies show that the more people are alike in their personality traits and come from similar homes and backgrounds, the more likely they are to stay together over time. There is logic in this; after all, life is a journey of challenges and confrontations, and the more that people are similar to each other in terms of the way they deal with crises, solve problems and make decisions, the more likely they will have, relatively speaking, fewer conflicts along the way. In the end, we get along best with ourselves and understand ourselves most. Maybe evolution wants diversity, but the mind wants to stay with the familiar. Sometimes intense flames of passion go out as quickly as they were ignited, whereas a relationship that is built slowly, brick by brick, lasts a long time.

Learning to Love and Create a Lasting, Oxytocin-Rich Relationship

When we find the one, or at least the one who is better than anyone who came along before, it's time to realize that from this moment biology and the wiring in our brains are working against us. Our genes do not encourage us to love for life, but to attract diversity. As evolved social mammals, we have every evolutionary reason to fail to form a lifelong, sexually monogamous relationship. This is because, in conditions of abundance, monogamy does not present a significant genetic survival advantage. Therefore, exchanging rings, signing the marriage register and making vows in front of family and friends are all very nice, but there is no guarantee that love will prevail. The sexual saturation effect, the Coolidge effect, will kick in sooner or later and the excitement will fade. And if that's not enough, pregnancy, births and raising children are not particularly compatible with marital libido.

So, then, what can be done?

In order to preserve love under these conditions, we need to create a relationship rich in oxytocin and not give up for a moment on the creation of the ingredients from which love is made. Professor Ruth Feldman from Bar-Ilan University followed new couples from the beginning of their relationship for over a year, periodically measuring the level of oxytocin in their blood. She measured the increase in the level of oxytocin while the subjects looked at pictures or videos of their partners. Thinking about our partner or seeing images of them immediately causes the release of oxytocin into the blood – if we still love them, of course. Feldman saw that for couples whose oxytocin levels remained high six months into their relationship, their chances of staying together until the end of the year were better, while for couples whose oxytocin level was lower when looking at pictures of their partner, the chances of breaking up were higher.

Oxytocin is the stuff of which partnerships are made. It's a good exercise to look at a picture of your partner and notice which emotions arise. If positive feelings of affection and warmth ensue, this is of course a sign of love, but if negative feelings of stress, pressure or distress arise, it may be time to go for counselling or even consider a breakup. Emotions drive our behaviour, and if those emotions are negative, the state of the relationship may worsen – and there is no reason for us to be unhappy with each other.

Oxytocin, the love hormone, is what connects us and turns us from strangers into lovers. At the end of the falling in love phase, which, as mentioned, can last from six hours to two years, but on average lasts a year, two things can happen: a decline in excitement and increased distancing until the couple part, or a stable bond of friendship and trust. To continue to maintain a stable bond of true friendship and trust in real life, after those butterflies in the stomach have gone quiet, and worries and obligations build up, you mustn't stop creating oxytocin for a moment. Oxytocin is the glue that creates the bond, and without it, the bond will be broken and you revert to being strangers. Remember that since there are no family ties between you – you don't share genes and you haven't grown up together since childhood – your relationship depends even more on the love hormone that you produce during your life together.

Since the lifetime of oxytocin in the blood is only six minutes, here is a prescription to help preserve it . . .

Look deeply into your partner's eyes, for at least 30 seconds
Do this while talking, when naked, during sex and when you want to know how your partner feels. The eyes are a window to the emotional brain and looking into them causes an immediate release of oxytocin and the activation of the vagus nerve, the relaxation system. Eye contact is important for increasing empathy, synchronizing brainwaves, and a sense of closeness.

Hold hands
When you hold hands, oxytocin is released, and coordination ensues in the breathing rate, heart rate, and patterns of brain activity that contribute to pain reduction and relaxation. Hold hands, especially when one of you is stressed or in pain. I recommended hand-holding with your fingers intertwined, this being the best grip for showing passion and mutual attraction. If you don't feel comfortable holding hands, this is a strong signal of a bad relationship. Pay attention and check for a possible reason.

Plenty of touching, hugging and caressing
Stroke each other's hair, face, hands, arms and shoulder blades. You should touch while talking, when you meet, when you eat together, when you casually get up from the table and certainly when you get into bed at the end of the day and on waking. There are not enough words to emphasize the power of a warm hug to reduce tension, strengthen your relationship and increase confidence in it. Just as we are willing to reach out to a dog or cat when they need to be petted, so too does a human need to be touched. Hugs are just as important. I recommend you hug for at least 20 seconds, morning and evening. Oxytocin is released after a long hug just like it is when we are babies. A hug evokes positive feelings of presence (*someone supports me*), comfort, security and reciprocity. It is good for mental and physical health, activates the vagus nerve (for relaxation) and strengthens bonds.

Smile and laugh together

While smiling, muscles in the corners of our mouth and ears are put to work, sending a message to the brain to release serotonin, which improves the mood and induces relaxation. Smiling and laughing also activate the mirror neurons and will make your partner smile and laugh automatically, even if they are stressed or angry. There is nothing like smiling and laughing to reduce tension and end fights. We also bond more with those who make us laugh and smile, since laughter releases oxytocin and also boosts activity in the memory areas of the brain by 30 per cent.

Share five compliments a day

Compliments trigger a release of oxytocin. They miraculously improve relationships and contribute to closeness and generosity. We all want to be appreciated, especially by our partners. It's important to maintain a ratio of five compliments and positive statements for every criticism: for example, "I'm glad to see you", "Thank you for . . .", "You look great", and, "What you did/said made me more relaxed and happy." We need to remember the importance of compliments and kind words, precisely because we have a natural tendency toward negativity, focusing on what is bad instead of the good.

Share and listen to each other at least once a day

We all need to be seen and listened to with empathy, without judgement and without being offered advice. The people who listen to us and with whom we can share what we are going through are the people with whom we bond, thanks to the oxytocin that is released during heartfelt and empathic conversations. If we are able to share regularly with each other what we are going through, while listening to each other, we will become good friends and our libido will also increase. It is vulnerability and empathy that creates intimacy, especially in women. A woman's sexual arousal passes through the brain's centres of communication and emotion. The oxytocin released during an emotional and empathic conversation also stimulates the genitals. The love hormone is the orgasm hormone, and to reach orgasm you have to go through the emotional centres and stimulate the release of oxytocin. When we allow ourselves to be vulnerable, we also encourage the other party to be vulnerable, creating a strong sense of intimacy.

But when we feel that we cannot truly share what we are going through, and even hide these experiences, this can be a sign of a deterioration in a relationship which may, of course, also harm intimacy and sex. It is impossible to separate these things; hence the importance of practising active listening, especially in this age of inattention. Ask your partner how they feel, what are they going through, and how their day was. Remember to give them your full attention, make eye contact, focus on what your partner is saying, nod and make small comments. Do not judge, do not criticize and do not give advice. Listening is not the same as agreeing; you can listen fully to your partner's point of view without agreeing with it. Each of us has an entire emotional world that our partner is not necessarily a part of. When we go through things by ourselves, we usually feel worse and burden ourselves with feelings of guilt, self-blame and frustration. When we allow our partner a glimpse into our inner emotional world, this creates deep connections and attachment. This is, of course, in the form of a conversation between your emotions that doesn't take place out loud. Speech contributes to an increase in cortisol, the stress hormone, because it reminds us of all the things we haven't taken care of and have been assigned to our endless to-do list.

Listen to music and dance together

Music causes the release of oxytocin, so when enjoying music together, we connect and bond, especially when it's music we both love and which evokes pleasant memories. The music that releases the most oxytocin is the music we heard when we were young, around the age of 16, when the level of oxytocin being released is at its highest. In addition to listening to music from our teens, it's very important to dance. When we dance, making eye contact and touching while moving to the music, the brain releases a huge dose of oxytocin and our movements synchronize. When a couple dances, they form a wordless connection, reducing tension and creating contact that is full of warmth and love. Synchronization in the body will also affect synchronization in the mind. Dance lessons are a great gift for newlyweds.

Learn your love language and that of your partner

Each of us speaks a different language of love, a language shaped by those who raised us. Similar to our mother tongue, this language of love – whose patterns feel comfortable and natural to us – has been shaped by the stimulation we received from our parents. The common forms in which we received oxytocin from our parents formed our leading love language. Each of us has a primary language and a secondary language. According to bestselling author Gary Chapman, there are five love languages: words of affirmation, physical touch, quality time, acts of service and gift-giving. For a happy long-term relationship, we have to find out what our main love language is and what our partner's main love language is. Our partner grew up in a different environment, experienced different love stimuli and his or her mind was very likely shaped differently. The way we received love often shapes how we show love and expect to receive it.

- **Words of affirmation:** a person may feel loved when they hear words of affection and love, words of support, listening, empathy and encouragement. It is important for these people to hear words of affirmation in order to be assured of their partner's love.
- **Physical touch:** these people feel loved when touched. Kissing, hugging, caressing, holding hands – every form of touch is an expression of love for them and this is how they also show love.
- **Shared quality time:** this person will feel loved when quality time is spent with them, when we devote time to them and listen to what they are going through. The main thing is to do something together.
- **Acts of service:** this person feels loved when we do something for them or help them carry out their tasks. Take the car to the garage, wash dishes, cook or do the laundry, and vice versa – if they do any act of service for us, they are showing love.
- **The language of gifts:** this person feels loved when they receive a gift. No matter what kind of gift, the main thing is that the giver thought about it and expressed it. This individual shows love in the same way – either by making or buying gifts.

Knowing and using the right love language is essential for healthy communication. So much misunderstanding and heartache can be caused if we insist on communicating in our own natural love language, when the other person needs something completely different. There can be immense frustration on all sides. Sometimes you have to negotiate the languages of love in order to maintain a good relationship. It's important to remember this, because one of the strongest biases in our brain is "self-bias"; we are sure that other people are just like us – think like us, react like us, need the same things and have the same worldview.

Experiencing excitement together

Whether it's travelling together in the Himalayas, skydiving, visiting an amusement park or bungee jumping, from time to time do something with your partner that raises your levels of adrenaline (the thrill and survival hormone). When we are afraid or excited and our adrenaline is pumping, this affects the memory areas of the brain and, when combined with oxytocin, which is also released when we are frightened, creates a positive shared memory of something that makes us both feel good. Exciting and scary shared experiences help to strengthen the relationship bond.

A romantic dinner and making memories

Once a week sit down for a romantic meal with foods that increase libido, such as meat (but not too much), fish and seafood, chocolate, chilli, strawberries, almonds, pumpkin seeds, watermelon and honey. Fast food with a high fat content damages the libido. To reduce stress during and after the meal, try to avoid talking about the day you've had or the children. It's better to use your time together to share old memories, which stimulate oxytocin, by recalling trips taken together and events from the early days of your relationship. Looking at old photos and videos is another good way of sharing memories.

Having a weekly heart-to-heart conversation

Much of the time our conversation takes the form of updates: who did what, how, when and why. This type of communication does not bring people closer and may even create tension. An emotion-driven conversation about feelings, thoughts and what is really important to you is a much better way of connecting. Every now and then, try to have a soulful conversation, a deep and meaningful discussion about what you are going through and where your priorities lie. Open up about things that interest and intrigue you. In chapter 2, we looked at Professor Arthur Aron's questionnaire, which is designed to help strangers connect and fall in love. His 36 questions are about what motivates us, our relationships with our parents, our good and bad memories, what we value most and our dreams. Of course, these are questions that promote oxytocin production in the respondent. In order to fall in love with our partner again, it's important to have these sorts of meaningful conversations from time to time and not just endless routine small talk.

21 orgasms a month

The highest level of the love hormone is released during orgasm, which is why the frequency of our orgasms can directly affects the strength of our relationship. We are creatures designed to reproduce, and our brains are rewarded when we try. During orgasm, as previously mentioned, a link is formed in the brain between the pleasure and reward system (dopamine) and the attachment and love system (oxytocin). The brain associates our loved one with pleasure and produces dopamine when we see, smell or hear them. We learned that the recommendation for men is 21 orgasms monthly, due to the structure of the male reproductive system, and that the average man thinks about sex five times more than a woman does. Many men will say that their primary love language is touch. Part of empathy in a relationship can mean understanding that we are not built exactly the same as our partner and that we sometimes have different needs and desires. Much of the tension between spouses can arise from an incompatibility between the sexual needs of them both, which is why it is important to talk about this and not sweep it under the carpet. It's important to talk about our sexuality, what we like and what we don't like and what's good for us, and also ask for help if there are things that upset one of the partners and harm the sexual relationship.

Put phones away during quality time

We live in a very challenging age for oxytocin. The smartphones and the apps that have infiltrated our lives, the Skinner boxes of the 21st century, are programmed to deny our brains rest until we answer a message, read our notifications or respond to an email. They shorten our attention span, reduce eye contact with our partners and elevate stress – three factors that are deadly for any relationship. Studies show that in couples where one is glued to a cell phone while they are together, the likelihood of them separating increases by 30 per cent. The use of cell phones leads to less oxytocin and more upset in relationships.

Professor Sherry Turkle from MIT studies a common occurrence which does a lot of harm in marriages, both between partners and to their relationship with their children. She calls this "the elsewhere effect"; or, in other words, being alone together. We are in the same space, in the living room, in the restaurant or in bed, but each of us is lost in our cell phone. During this sort of "elsewhere time", Terkle saw a reduction in endorphins and oxytocin in both partners. We saw in an earlier chapter how an Israeli study in honour of Family Day 2018 found that a third of Israeli couples communicate only via WhatsApp. The rise in the level of oxytocin in the blood following the receipt of an emoji on WhatsApp is minimal, and therein lies the danger to the relationship. In our digital age, we need to develop a greater awareness of the serious consequences of less oxytocin flowing in our relationships.

Expand your circle of friends

Make friends with other couples – the relationship between couples who have a common social circle of friends is stronger. A group of couples who share meals, outings and experiences can contribute to strengthening your own partnership. Besides the fact that we are social beings who need a variety of social contacts, in addition to what each partner can provide, being with other couples allows us to examine our relationship in comparison to theirs and to talk about them in a manner that actually encourages us to talk about ourselves and our own relationship, in ways we might otherwise find difficult.

The love hormone is the critical ingredient for maintaining a long-term relationship. It's very easy to get carried away in the routine of our daily lives, to neglect our relationship, and for us to drift further and further apart without noticing. If falling in love happens in a turbulent and loud chemical storm, breaking up often happens slowly and quietly. The opposite of love is not hate but indifference. When the sight, sound, touch and smell of the partner no longer evoke anything, no electrical stimulation and no chemical response, this can be a sign that the love has dried up. To avoid this, you have to invest in the relationship and in the continued creation of the love hormones.

Make love part of your routine

To improve the foundations of a relationship, I recommended making the following actions part of your routine:

- Go for a walk and breathe clean air.
- Linger in the sunshine among trees and green vegetation.
- Pet the dog or cat.
- Spend time with friends and tell them how much they mean to you.
- Exchange compliments with your loved one.
- Cue up the playlist you like, close your eyes and connect to the music.
- Dance, together or alone, to the music you heard when you were 16.
- Do some physical activity with the one you love.
- Laugh until your stomach hurts.

- Sit with the one you love, look in their eyes, hold hands and say three compliments to each other.
- Make love slowly and gently, pleasure yourself and connect with feelings.
- Prepare a nutritious meal with foods that increase oxytocin production, such as figs, avocado, watermelon, bananas, spinach, green tea, almonds and pumpkin seeds.

How to Beat the Coolidge Effect and Keep the Sexual Excitement

While multiple orgasms are important for the production of oxytocin and deepening the relationship, the downside is an acceleration of the onset of the Coolidge effect, the state of sexual saturation. As with the mice and rats, the same stimulation over time leads to tolerance and feelings of boredom. From sexual encounter to sexual encounter, over the years, more and more stimulation is needed for us to reach orgasm with the same partner. The Coolidge effect is a fact of life and we cannot change that. Any new stimulus will always be more intriguing and exciting than what we have known for years. Evolution has wired our brains to encourage genetic diversity.

So, are we prisoners of our genes, and every connection is doomed to fail because of the Coolidge effect? I really don't think so. We are neither mice nor chimpanzees; we are human beings with a developed prefrontal cortex, which allows us to see things as they are, to explore and learn about ourselves. We have the option to choose what we do with this knowledge. In my opinion, understanding the way our brain is wired allows us first and foremost to free ourselves from the inhibitions of guilt and shame, which erode relationships. We must accept that this is our biology and it is completely natural and normal for any couple to experience a decline in sexual attraction and excitement over time. That way, we will be freed from the automatic need to apportion blame or to start thinking that our partner is actually unsuitable for us. Understanding the biology of our sexuality, which drives us into the arms of others, can help us to break free from the shackles, and to be much more authentic and open about our sexuality and sexual needs.

For generations we have been taught to hide our sexuality, to be ashamed of it, and not to talk about it. We pass on a lot of these inhibitions about sex from one generation to the next. It's time to break free from all these boundaries and misconceptions about love and sex, accept ourselves as we are and develop healthier love lives as a result. It's important to understand that what stimulates and turns us on is in the prehistoric part of the brain, far below the new part – the realm of political correctness. Allow yourself to be authentic and talk openly with your partner about what turns you on and stimulates you. Introduce plenty of variety in the bedroom through role-playing, interesting sex toys, bondage and games of domination, if that appeals to you. Watch erotic films – either alone or together. The need to maintain a satisfactory long-term sex life is not always obvious and requires a lot of investment.

As we have seen, men think more about sex and usually admit to needing more frequent intercourse than women do. When the divide in their sexual needs is too great in a couple, frustration and resentment can accumulate over the years. It's important to talk things out and rank sex as a priority no less important than all the other issues you discuss and negotiate. Things that are not talked about in the bedroom will emerge in everyday life as fights, jealousies, bitterness, cynicism and the like. If one of the partners feels unattractive or even rejected and sexually unwanted, these feelings will not stay in the bedroom and can lead to many tensions in the relationship. A lot of the quarrels between spouses have their roots in the bedroom. Sex at least once a week increases the level of happiness in a relationship, according to reports from people living in long-term relationships.

How to settle the contradiction? After all, in order to maintain a happy relationship, you need to have a lot of sex, but after a long time together, the desire for sex decreases due to the Coolidge effect. First, let's recognize that this really is a fundamental contradiction, and if we add to it the stress of everyday life, work and children, it becomes a monumental challenge. In my opinion, this contradiction is one of the main causes of breakups. Desire decreases over time, we make countless excuses, and slowly we move further and further away from each other and the emotional connection lessens.

What is the solution? The solution is to place our sex life at the centre of our relationship, just like all our other shared concerns. We have a tendency to push sex to the bottom of our list of priorities, doing it only if there is some time and energy left at the end of the day. We don't discuss it and we don't live the oxytocin life anymore. It is important to understand that a situation where nothing happens in the bedroom for weeks and even entire months is like having serious leaks in the plumbing of your house. The leaks will eventually destroy the foundations. Now, it wouldn't occur to us to ignore a leaking pipe; we would take action to protect our home. So why do we neglect our sex lives?

There can be several reasons for this, and all of them require care and attention. If the lack of desire results from anger and negative emotions we have accumulated, they will not disappear but only worsen if we do not create positive emotions as well. That's why, before it's too late, we need to break down the anger, discuss what's bothering us, talk about our needs and get outside help. There is no couple in the world who would not benefit from counselling. I believe that if relationship counselling were available as part of our basic health care, physical and mental illnesses would decline significantly in the population of adults and children alike.

In some instances, the reasons for a lack of desire don't stem from unresolved mutual anger, but mainly from the Coolidge effect combined with stress. The stress hormone, cortisol, causes a significant decrease in libido, which spirals into a vicious cycle. We are stressed, our desire decreases, and we no longer desire to touch or make love, so less oxytocin is produced, leading to even more stress . . . and so the cycle continues.

Therefore, if we do feel emotionally overwhelmed and mentally tired, due to difficulties at work or from child raising, it's important to re-centre ourselves. We need to find ways to relax, shed some of the load, rest, ask for help with tasks, delegate, make time for ourselves, switch off phones, and make regular appointments for reflexology, massage, acupuncture or any other stress-relieving treatment. Get out into nature, engage in physical activity and enjoy music. It's important to maintain your emotional health so that you are available for love.

A combination of stress and the Coolidge effect can cause any relationship to collapse. Libido is a momentary and deceptive feeling that changes all the time, depending on the chemicals in the body. If we wait for an erotic charge to hit us like a lightning bolt, giving us the sudden urge to make love on the kitchen counter (like before), it simply won't happen. We may have to be proactive about stimulating desire, warming up the engines and producing sex chemicals through soft (or strong) touch, sex toys (there's a wide variety available today), sex videos, massage with warm oil, sexy music and – whoop! – the sexual brain awakens, we get down to business and enjoy a surge of endorphins, serotonin, testosterone, oxytocin, phenethylamine and dopamine straight to the brain. Straightaway, we feel calmer, more connected, and sleep then follows.

It is important to note that penetration is not necessary and neither is orgasm. Human sexuality is a broad and fascinating field of knowledge. The world of tantra and the other arts of love provide couples with wonderful tools to improve their sex life and achieve satisfying and emotional connections full of oxytocin. Today, there are also virtual courses that can make lots of excellent exercises available to you from the comfort of your double bed. If you've never been taught to make love and to get to know your sexuality, now is the time. Do whatever you like together; the main thing is to produce oxytocin in the bedroom. Don't let stress and the Coolidge effect triumph.

Along with prioritizing your sex life and love, it's also important to give each other space and to do things separately. Following the initial mouse experiment that proved the Coolidge effect, the researchers separated the male and female for a week; the animals then treated each other as if they had met for the first time and orgasm rapidly ensued. In other words, sometimes our brain needs a break, some distance and for longing to have time to develop, to perform a kind of reboot that will stir up excitement again. "Together and separately" – this mantra sits at the core of a healthy relationship: doing things together and tending to your love life, while each of you also gets to enjoy your own independence, desires, ambitions and authenticity. It's important to continue doing things apart, alone or with friends, to maintain your own hobbies and enjoy your personal circles of friends.

Interestingly, the "Nida" period practised in Judaism tallies with these findings. During Nida, from the time of menstruation until ovulation, a couple avoids sexual contact, thus creating a distance that reduces the Coolidge effect and contributes to renewed sexual excitement toward the partner. Studies done on couples enjoying their "second time around", a new relationship created out of the wreckage of failed partnerships, similarly showed that those who decide not to cohabit manage to sustain their initial passion for longer. The biological explanation is the resulting longing and the milder exposure to a partner's stimuli. The higher the exposure and the longer you are together, the sooner the Coolidge effect will set in.

However, so-called "second marriages" are 70 per cent more likely to break up, lasting an average of two years. This happens for a couple of reasons. One is the negative, unprocessed past experiences that we carry with us into the new relationship, which may have consequences for our new partner. We don't really learn from our past experiences, and bring along a stack of concerns and fear of further harm. Another reason is that the relationship may be technically more complex and affected by various external factors. Our brains also become less flexible as we get older. The habits we have created over the years become entrenched in our minds, and any attempt to "move our cheese" is met with more resistance.

Because of all these reasons, it's important to navigate a second relationship with great care, staying aware of the difficulties and avoiding potential pitfalls. For example, don't rush to move in together, bringing along all of your kids from your previous relationships. First, because of the Coolidge effect, which will certainly not help the challenges faced in your new partnership. Second, because confrontations with any new family members may intensify your relationship conflicts. Remember, the selfish gene will always make us put the needs of those children who share our genes before the needs of genes from another source.

Sex is not the exclusive preserve of young people. During our lives, there is a decrease in the production of sex hormones that affects the strength of sexual desire in women, while a decrease in oestrogen causes vaginal dryness. However, today women and men are much more aware of the importance of maintaining a sex life throughout their life and are willing to use preparations and aids to overcome any physiological limitations. In a survey conducted in the US among women and men between the ages of 60 and 80, about 90 per cent of the men and 70 per cent of the women stated that they had enjoyed sex in the past year. Additionally, 62 per cent of women and 86 per cent of men rated sex as "important to very important" for maintaining a relationship in their golden years. Sexual activity contributes to the longevity of the brain. During sexual activity and orgasm, whether together or separately, during masturbation, the activity in various areas of the brain is greatly increased, causing regeneration and renewal. Every day we lose some neurons in the brain, and brain activity during sex or masturbation can cause regeneration and help repair the damage resulting from stress.

Diet also affects libido and there are certain foods that help stimulate lust, so adding them to your diet can boost your levels of desire. Avocado, asparagus and bananas provide the bromelain enzymes, improving erectile function. Pomegranate juice helps to increase testosterone levels. Spicy peppers invigorate the blood and raise the body temperature. Eat radish for that sharp tingling on the tongue. Caviar is rich in zinc and helps produce testosterone. Garlic stimulates the blood and increases alertness. And don't forget chocolate, which contains phenethylamine to create a feeling of euphoria, and lastly almonds, an ancient symbol of fertility, rich in vitamin E and magnesium.

Argue Properly and Create a Low-Cortisol Relationship

Just as it's crucial to keep up the production of the materials from which love is made in order to maintain a relationship bond, it's also important to reduce, if possible, the materials that create hatred. Every time we attack, insult, criticize, blame, judge, humiliate, despise or treat each other with cynicism and sarcasm, higher amounts of the stress hormones, cortisol and adrenaline, are secreted. Arguments that usually start over something trivial can easily degenerate into a rash of accusations and insults, doubling and tripling the cortisol level of the initial argument.

It seems to be impossible to live without fighting. Ninety per cent of tiffs are long-running recurrences, and 70 per cent of fights between couples have no solution at all. They arise from differences in attitude and are often a means for releasing tension and a desperate call for attention. If we recall Professor Sapolsky's research with baboons, an integral part of our self-calming mechanism when we are stressed is to "take it out on someone else". Since we can't take it out on our boss and shouldn't take it out on our children, those in the line of fire are nearly always our partners.

However, quarrels can indicate a healthy relationship. If we sometimes fight, this means we are able to tell each other what bothers us, what our limits are, and that we feel secure enough in our relationship to express anger, a very basic and important emotion. In a partnership where no one fights, there is the likelihood that something is being suppressed, that one of you is feeling resentful, or, on the other hand, completely indifferent. A healthy and stable relationship stems from a couple's ability to manage their conflicts, deal with personal and joint stress and create a reasonable balance between negative gestures (cortisol gestures) and positive gestures (oxytocin gestures) in the relationship. Since 95 per cent of our communication is emotional, and we affect each other's emotions through our mirror neurons, it is important to manage cortisol and adrenaline during a fight. Without anger management, the stress hormones will automatically escalate the conflict, push all the anger buttons and worsen the relationship. This is why it is very important to learn "how to fight correctly" with the help of the following guide:

1. Avoid casting aspersions

Releasing pressures and unloading tension on our partner will nearly always involve casting aspersions, which we could also call "projections". Oftentimes we're not actually fighting with our partner as such, but struggling with other things from our own past or present, or with characteristics of ourselves that we don't like.

There is no one who can push all our buttons like our partner can, because they show us different aspects of ourselves that we struggle with; for better or worse, they act as our mirror. Mostly, we are not angry at all about what we think is angering us, but simply casting aspersions: we take a negative characteristic of ourselves, mainly about unresolved things from our past, and project this on to the other person or into a situation. When we do this kind of projecting, we convince ourselves that a particular emotion or issue that comes up is the other person's and not ours.

Projection is actually a self-defence mechanism, designed to protect us from negative emotions, stress and coping with trauma. Projection is the opposite of vulnerability and it surfaces when our feelings cause us discomfort, nervousness, embarrassment or are related to a trauma we have experienced. When these feelings arise, we look for a quick way to get rid of them, and the oldest and fastest trick is to blame someone else. The five most common forms of human speech, as observed in different languages, are:

1. condescending/arguing
2. attacking
3. blaming
4. obedience
5. talking

Note that only one of these approaches produces dialogue. Our automatic form of communication is aggressive and full of aspersions, and when we are under pressure and stressed, the attacks, blaming and projections increase, resulting in a fight or flight response. It is difficult, almost impossible, to engage in dialogue and empathetic discourse when we are stressed, and the worse the stress, the more violent our communication will be. This is why fights often escalate within minutes, especially the more we carry unresolved hurt. In most cases, these automatic defence mechanisms will cause us to project our negative feelings on to our partners.

How do we know when we are just casting aspersions? Every relationship has its share of tension, disappointments and disagreements. Disagreements are healthy; they show that we are both independent people with our own needs and desires. However, when couples feel that they are emotionally overwhelmed and focus only on the faults of the other party, and when conflicts become routine, it is time to stop and take a closer look. What is happening to you? Maybe you are casting aspersions?

- **If you find yourself complaining** all the time about your partner, take a moment to look within, at how you feel about yourself. The flaws you constantly find in your partner . . . can you also find them in some way in yourself?
- **Do you blame your partner** for how they make you feel, or for anything negative that happens to you? The first step to a healthy and supportive relationship is to accept personal responsibility for your own stress and the emotions you feel, and to break the toxic cycle of blame.
- **Your past is not your future** – you do have a choice. Often, during an argument, we are not reacting to something that is happening now, but to events from the past, which we project onto this moment. Situations we've already experienced, emotions we've already felt, and vulnerabilities we've already been hurt by, we repeat them again and again. Our psyche is made up of the sum of all our past experiences. It isn't easy to let go of the past. So we need to free ourselves from entire belief systems and the conditioning created in our brains as a result of the negative things that have happened to us. This conditioning consists of many generalities. For example, we project onto our partner everything we think about men/women, based on our past experiences, or even the experiences of people close to us, whose pain we shared. Projecting a negative belief system onto your partner, following a previous trauma, results in a vicious cycle of reliving that trauma every day. Therefore, when a conflict arises, instead of succumbing to the reptilian brain's automatic response, we have to pause a moment, activate the prefrontal cortex and examine our response. The current situation can bring up feelings from the past, which is what the brain is supposed to do. Recognize these feelings for what they are and share them with your partner. They don't know what happened or what you are going through. Try to explain to your partner, "When you act like this, I feel fear/frustration/guilt/sadness/anger/horror, because it reminds me of . . . I want you to be aware of that." That way, you will start to get to know each other better and be more empathetic. Remember, everyone experiences crises and difficulties. Allow yourself to be vulnerable, to slowly open the box of traumas from the past. This will only bring you closer, take a weight off your shoulders and bind you together. We are supposed to help each other. People naturally want

to help and facilitate, certainly when it comes to their loved ones. So give them a chance.

Aspersions can destroy any relationship. The automatic defence mechanisms our brain produces in times of stress and crisis reduce our ability to empathize and increase aggressiveness and the need to blame. In order to succeed in our relationships, we must learn to argue properly, reduce cortisol and try to see in every conflict an opportunity to learn more about ourselves and our partner. It's an opportunity to learn more about precisely the things that we consciously try so hard to hide and repress, which erupt during a fight. Why did we react that way? What are the feelings that a certain behaviour triggers in us? What are the emotions we feel during the argument? Where do they come from? What is the conditioning that creates our reaction and what will make us feel better? Our partners are a mirror of us and we mirror them; they will sometimes be a source of pain, but they can also be the best medicine.

2. Avoid idle threats

Threatening to leave is a doomsday weapon, since it undermines the security of the relationship. Even in moments of overwhelming anger, avoid using it. A threat to leave makes the couple think about "the day after" – and that's not what you meant. As we know, each of us is programmed to put ourselves first, to protect our self-image, to survive and reproduce successfully. Most of the time the brain is not in the here and now, but is busy predicting the future. As soon as someone brings up the possibility of splitting up, the minds of both partners are already producing a simulation of what life will look like after separation. A threat to leave can lead to the conclusion that there is no longer any point in investing in a relationship that depends on restraint. Depending on the extent to which your partner has abandonment anxiety based on past experiences, their mind will enter survival mode and all their conditioning will go into overdrive.

3. Eliminate the "four horsemen of the apocalypse" from your quarrels

Relationship researcher Dr John Gottman analysed more than 3,000 15-minute fights between married couples. He tracked facial expressions, vocal tones, eye contact, intonation, transcripts of conversations, and asked the couples to complete questionnaires. He focused on the emotional expressions of each of the spouses, and how each experienced the other's feelings. He included additional information about their stress levels by measuring their heart rate, skin conductance and blood flow. From his research on quarrels, Gottman was able to predict with 90 per cent accuracy whether couples would stay together or break up based on a 15-minute argument, no matter what it was about. Gottman found four patterns of communication that predict a breakup. He called them "the four horsemen", and they are:

Criticism: "You're always so selfish"; "you're just like your mother"; "you don't care . . ." This is not about the targeted criticism of a particular issue or specific behaviour, which we would like to see changed, but a strong criticism of the partner's own character, which usually results, as mentioned, from casting aspersions. A toxic criticism is a message that is worded in a way that implies something is flawed in the partner, their personality and character. Such a message will provoke a negative reaction in any healthy individual. The person will feel attacked and fight back. Instead of criticizing the other party, try to express your needs in a matter-of-fact and specific manner, without harming your partner's personality and self-image. A person with a healthy self-image can shrug off personal criticism as part of their normal self-defence mechanisms. The antidote to criticism is to speak in the first person – "I feel . . ." – and to praise them.

Contempt: *What an idiot; you are such a loser* . . . Insults, ridicule, condescension, derogatory names, curses, disdainful imitation and disrespectful gestures, such as eye rolling, as well as cynicism and sarcasm . . . contempt is expressed not only in words but also in the tone of voice, facial expressions and body language. Most of us have a harder time with grimaces and body language. The purpose of contempt is to make the other party feel worthless, and it blocks real communication and problem-solving. This type of communication is the strongest predictor of breakup and produces the highest level of cortisol. To change this pattern, you have to absolutely agree to avoid mockery, insults, cynicism and any other form of contempt. The antidotes to contempt are mutual respect, gestures of appreciation and recognition of the good in the partner. If you can't succeed at this, if you feel a lack of appreciation for your partner and you can't find what attracted you to them in the first place, it's time to separate. There's no point in continuing to make each other miserable; the price is too high for both body and soul.

Defensiveness: when we are attacked, we defend ourselves, repel the blows and strike back: *I'm not responsible for us being late, it's because of you; I'm not angry, you're the one who interprets my every reaction like that.* Defending ourselves by claiming innocence can make the other party feel as if their words have not been taken seriously or even considered. In a healthy relationship, we should always strive for validation. Validate your partner's words, giving them space and consideration, instead of automatically pushing them away. For example, instead of, "What happened? I didn't raise my voice, that's your interpretation," try, "I hear what you're saying, I may have raised my voice and I apologize if you felt bad." If you notice that you always tend toward defensiveness, you don't have to respond immediately. You can tell your partner that you listened to what he or she said, and that you want to give it some thought when you are calmer. Remember, each of us needs to be listened to, validated, understood and appreciated. The antidotes to defensiveness are to accept even a modicum of responsibility for the issue your partner raised.

Stonewalling: this involves escape, seclusion or emotional withdrawal, such as when the person with whom you are having an argument shuts down and runs away. They don't respond verbally but only with their body language, including thunderous silences, folding their arms while avoiding eye contact, leaving the room, turning on the TV and shunning contact. You are left feeling your partner is dug in behind a wall and there is no way to reach them. This happens when the other person feels emotionally overwhelmed and it's their way of dealing with the situation. They usually didn't choose this response consciously; it's the reptilian brain, the amygdala at work. Their thoughts revolve around the injustice done to them, the justification of their actions and the blame they can attach to the other party. In this situation, the other party feels ignored, there is no validation, there is no understanding and the quarrel usually escalates in an attempt to engage their partner in some kind of interaction.

The antidote to being stonewalled is to agree in advance to a ceasefire whenever these situations arise. Decide on a timeout of at least 20 minutes (the lifetime of cortisol in the blood) before talking about the subject again. It's very important to give time and space to yourself and your partner, especially in stressful situations.

We can see that, just as different people speak different love languages, there are also different stress languages. Different people react differently in stressful situations. Our emotional systems are formed in the first few years of our life and are a product of genetics and epigenetics, the environment in which we grew up and the people who raised us. It can be difficult to change the shape of our emotional systems, so it's up to us to recognize our languages, our way of coping with stressful situations, to talk with our partner and ask for understanding. Since all of our stress languages – fight, flight, freeze or tend and befriend, aka fawning – have a high potential to increase conflict, we must consciously learn nonviolent forms of communication. We must learn to communicate differently. Otherwise, the automatic responses of the reptilian brain will drag us into a vicious cycle of cortisol-saturated relationship stress, which will eventually cause our brains to label our partner as someone we hate, someone to run from. The mere voice and appearance of our partner end up arousing fear and loathing instead of tenderness and love.

To prevent this, Gottman developed a formula for a healthy relationship based on a ratio of 1:5. For every dose of cortisol, get five doses of oxytocin. Five tender moments for each verbal blow. If we said something mean and unnecessary, we should create five positive interactions, preferably on the same day. In couples with a strong bond, Gottman noticed a ratio of 1:15 – 15 good moments for every negative one. This is something we can always fix if we want to, which is why we should consciously learn how to make up with each other and live in harmony.

4. Use nonviolent communication to properly manage the dispute

Most of the quarrels between spouses are repetitive and concern the same topics – the division of housework, money matters and the children's education. This is why, before losing control, giving in to automatic reactions and escalating the argument through attack, blame and condescension, try practising the following nonviolent communication steps for managing a fight:

First, say what you feel: since our automatic tendency is to blame, try to explain what you feel, why you are really angry, and what caused you to feel this way. Remember, emotions indicate a need. Our emotions represent an opportunity to understand what our needs are and learn from them. What unfulfilled need caused us to feel hurt and made us angry? It could be a sense of helplessness – because our partner doesn't understand us – that caused us to lose control. It is therefore important not to blame and attack but to explain what you feel and to evoke understanding in the other party. Do not shut down or retaliate. Focus on talking about "I" and not "you": *I feel that . . ., it hurts me that . . ., it scares me that . . .* The response you will receive will be completely different when you speak in "I" and not in "you", and during the quarrel, there'll be a meaningful connection and not a fistfight.

Listen to your partner: ignore the temptation to shut down and run away. Try to listen to and understand what your partner is attempting to relate. Look at your partner out of empathy, out of a desire to help them deal with their feelings. When we're angry we don't listen and it's hard for us to muster empathy; we focus instead on deflecting accusations and maintaining our positive self-image. Sometimes you may have to leave the argument for a moment, look at your partner from a distance, muster empathy and listen to their pain.

Ask: after you have explained what you feel and what your unmet needs are, and after you have listened to what your partner has to say, it's time to ask some questions. Ask your partner whatever it is you want them to do to fulfil your need and cancel those negative feelings. When we make demands, the other party often immediately shuts down, but when we genuinely ask for what we need, it can arouse in others the desire to help and support us, and doesn't provoke power struggles. After a clear and precise request, you can negotiate over the requests, feelings and needs of you both from a loving and supportive position.

The principles of nonviolent communication, or "compassionate communication", developed by Dr Marshall Rosenberg, are not to speak in terms of "accusations, criticisms and demands", but to speak in the language of "feelings, needs and requests" without judgement and without belittling: *What do I feel in this situation? What do I need? What am I asking for?*

There are basic needs common to all humans, which arouse strong emotions in us, and they are:

- food, sleep and sex
- security and financial certainty
- belonging, identity and love
- respect, understanding and appreciation
- self-fulfilment and freedom

Which of those needs do you need to ask about?

5. Always make up afterwards

Chimpanzee researcher Professor Frans de Waal, who followed the relationships within a group of chimpanzees for seven years, noticed something interesting. The strongest ties were not between individuals who didn't fight at all, but between individuals who fought often and reconciled regularly. Chimpanzees make up with each other through mutual lice removal and rubbing each other. De Waal saw that reconciliation is very important for strengthening the social bond. The same is true for us. No matter what the topic is, nor how long the quarrel lasts, it is always important to reconcile and not persist in anger. Within an hour and a half of the quarrel, it's a good idea to make up with each other and renew contact. A quarrel that doesn't end in reconciliation, but rather a quick return to routine as if nothing had happened, causes emotional disconnection and leaves negative debris in the relationship. Conversely, continuing to quarrel over days or weeks must also be completely avoided, because then the frustration, anger and resentment will only increase and it will be very difficult to reconcile afterwards.

However, healthy reconciliation should not spring from subservience, fear or the need to apologize for something you didn't do in order to gain peace. The absence of authenticity leads to a build-up of resentment that will eventually erupt.

Making up with each other means a return to the partnership and the ensuing oxytocin-producing gestures: a soft touch, kind words, asking for forgiveness and apologizing. Quarrels have a certain emotional dynamic. They can start as a volcanic eruption of strong, angry feelings, frustration and distress, the signals our needs are not being met, but once we have let off steam, said what bothers us, cried, bared our emotions, expressed our needs, the cortisol level drops and we feel more relaxed. This is the right time for gestures of reconciliation and renewing contact. It doesn't always happen to both partners at the same time; sometimes one person maintains a high cortisol level for much longer than the other. Therefore, after each quarrel, the partners should take turns in initiating the reconciliation to end the conflict. Oxytocin reconciliation gestures can include a hand on the shoulder, any kind of touch, an apology, a conciliatory smile, a humorous comment, a gesture of goodwill, a note of forgiveness, a kindness, a gift, preparing food or a supportive statement – anything positive. You should decide what your reconciliation gestures will be so that when one of you initiates them the other will respond and reconcile.

It's important to remember that forgiveness and apology do not make us weak or subservient, but the opposite. When we apologize and explain ourselves, talking about why we were offended, what hurt us and how we feel, this makes us more vulnerable and evokes empathy in our partner.

There are two types of forgiveness. One kind is to forgive those who hurt us and end the relationship. The second kind is to forgive those who hurt us and continue the relationship, hopefully even strengthening it through reconciliation and the creation of positive feelings. Both types of forgiveness contribute to our wellbeing and most moments of forgiveness between couples are of the second type, making these even more important. In terms of the body, refusing to forgive and harbouring negative emotions weakens our mental and physical health.

In 2013, Dr Pietro Pietrini from the University of Pisa in Italy performed MRI scans of brains while asking his participants to imagine scenarios with people close to them, who had hurt them in various ways, and to decide whether or not they forgave them or even sought revenge. The subjects rated the levels of anger and frustration they felt when they imagined the scenario, and then reported whether they forgave them or not. Pietrini found that in those who chose to forgive, their decision was linked to a positive emotional state and increased activity in the areas of the brain associated with empathy, intimacy, conscience and self-awareness.

The psychologist Dr Charlotte vanOyen-Witvliet examined what happens to the body during times of forgiveness. She reviewed data on blood pressure, heart rate, facial muscle tension, blood cortisol levels and skin perspiration in different people while they were thinking about someone who hurt them in the past while imagining themselves forgiving or reconciling with them, or remembering forgiveness if this had in fact occurred. VanOyen-Witvliet discovered that their stress levels increased while the subjects recalled the incidents, but returned to normal when they imagined themselves forgiving and making up.

To apologize and forgive. To communicate in respectful and kind ways without insults and humiliation. To be familiar with acts of reconciliation, the love languages and the stress languages of each other – these are critical skills for a stable, strong and healthy relationship.

Let's remember that each of us comes from a different nurturing environment, where our brains received different stimuli and we learned to communicate in a certain way, for better or for worse. This is what we bring to our relationships and we aren't even aware of it. It is not easy to change the languages and habits that have been wired into our minds through our family and a lifetime of experiences. But if there is anyone who can help us change the conditions that harm us, it could only be a partner who loves and wants to support us. In order to help each other we must share, allow ourselves to be vulnerable, get to know each other in the deepest way, without judgement and criticism, and develop relationship awareness. When the storm has passed, we should talk to each other about what happened to us, explain where it came from, and then we can continue on our journey together.

Couples who manage to communicate and make up with each other even after the most heated quarrels are more likely to stay together for a long time. If you find it difficult to reconcile, you should seek the help of a relationship therapist as soon as possible and prevent resentment and mutual hostility from mounting, which can, of course, be fatal to your relationship.

The bonobo monkeys can teach us about the importance of conciliatory love making. Their every fight and disagreement ends in mutual manual or oral pleasure and make-up sex. Sexual contact is perfect for immediately lifting levels of oxytocin, endorphins, serotonin and dopamine; and it follows that the stress markers then decline, improving the mood of both partners and strengthening their relationship. The problem is that sometimes the cortisol generated during a fight suppresses the libido, and because women have higher blood cortisol levels, it takes twice as long for them to relax or even think about sex. Maybe the solution is to fight naked? Take off your clothes and then argue – it will increase the levels of oxytocin and serotonin straightaway and the fight will then be calmer . . . !

6. Don't go to bed too angry

This is one piece of advice every young couple hears at the beginning of their journey together, and today there is a scientific explanation from the field of brain research. At night our brain doesn't rest for a moment; it paralyzes the reception of stimuli through the senses and stops sending messages to the muscles in order to invest in the business of processing. During sleep, the brain consolidates and fixes emotional memories. Emotions from the last few days are reconstructed along with all the stimuli related to them, what was good and what was bad, and memories are fixed according to the intensity of the emotion. Once the memories have been fixed, it's harder to suppress them.

So, if we spent the evening in a heated argument and went to sleep flooded with negative emotions, continuing the argument in our head until sleep overcomes us, there is little chance in the morning we will feel the desire to look into the eyes of our partner, hold hands and caress. At night, the brain processes the negative memories and associates them with stimuli from our partner – meaning that their appearance, voice and touch will become associated with an unpleasant memory instead. The partner is labelled as something negative, which makes us feel bad. The more difficult, painful and traumatic the quarrel, the more the brain will push us to escape into sleep, only to process these powerful emotional stimuli into memory. That's why it is very important in such situations not to go to sleep and to protect your hippocampus, the long-term memory area. Talk until two in the morning, if necessary, and try to reach a more empathetic conversation. Even if you don't completely make up with each other, try to go to bed on a reasonably positive note, feeling that you have heard each other out, that you understand and accept the feelings and needs of each other, that your relationship is strong and secure and that you will continue to work on it tomorrow because it is important to you. Unfortunately, sometimes after many years of frustrating fights, sleeping separately, sometimes for several nights and with a lot of brewing resentment, couples reach the point where the very sight and sound of their partner evokes irrational, sometimes unconscious negative feelings. In this situation, the positive influence of oxytocin diminishes, and breaking up becomes only a matter of time.

7. Use humour

Laughter is a universal language, connecting all members of the human race. Everyone can communicate with humour. One of the first qualities people say they look for in a partner is humour. Someone to make them laugh. Humour increases oxytocin, immediately activates the vagus nerve through the facial muscles, triggers relaxation and quickly reduces stress.

As we've seen, it's healthy to be funny or in the company of funny people. Humour makes things easier and allows us not to take ourselves or reality too seriously. Humour helps us to make up with each other by reducing stress and allowing tension to be released through laughter. Studies have shown that couples who laugh together stay together. Humour is also a communication channel, a way to break down barriers and create a more relaxed atmosphere. The humour channel makes it possible to broadcast messages or criticize in a way that will not provoke a hostile reaction from the other person, and might even promote listening. Humour is also a defence mechanism against anxiety: when you laugh at things they seem less threatening.

However, it's important to distinguish between different styles of humour, because certain styles such as sarcasm, aggressive humour and mockery don't contribute to a relationship. They only cause conflict to worsen under the onslaught of very negative feelings. Types of humour that contribute to a relationship are those that improve your mood, enable a more optimistic view and provide a positive perspective. Another helpful style of humour is when a couple can share jokes that both of them find funny and other amusing comments that bring them together.

Yet another style of humour is the ability to laugh at yourself, your own flaws, troubles and failures. Those who can do this develop a resistance to future setbacks. The ability to laugh at yourself is a highly effective defence mechanism; after all, who wants to attack a person who attacks himself?

8. Leave your family out of it

There are hardly any couples who don't argue over the issue of relations with their families of origin. For years, long before we met our partner, we maintained and probably still maintain an extensive and important relationship with our family of origin, which includes relationships with our mother, father, siblings, grandparents and extended family members, all bunched together and separately. The dynamics of the family system are varied, complex and often so deeply rooted that an outsider can find them difficult to understand. In this context, the partner is, and always will be, a stranger.

Family systems are very strong, and while the strength of those connections and their effect on a person varies, it's usually still there. From an evolutionary point of view, we appear to be programmed to protect and to preserve the strongest bonds with the people who share genes with us. Their success is our success and therefore this system is complex and interventional. Usually, the more that our families of origin differ from each other, the greater the friction and mutual misunderstanding. Countless partnerships have ended because of issues related to the families of origin. So it's important to consider these eternal axioms in advance:

- First, families of origin can never be objective on any subject. They are programmed to favour the offspring who carries their genes against all others.
- Second, the gene preservation law: there is no one in the world who is good enough for the offspring; that is, worthy of being included in the family gene pool.

That's why the best advice for preserving a harmonious relationship is under no circumstances to involve the families of origin in your quarrels. Do not ask for their advice, do not use them as a way to get things off your chest if they concern your partner, and do not use them as arbitrators or peacemakers. While the pair of you reconcile and curl up in bed together, flooded with oxytocin, they will stew in their bad thoughts and negative emotions about your partner – God forbid, not about you. When you feel the need to tell, vent or process your thoughts, call a friend instead. As an additional note, do not do to another family member what you would find hateful: never interfere in the marital relations of your children or your other family members.

The Female Brain and the Male Brain

"Men are from Mars, women are from Venus," said the popular marriage counselor and author John Gray – many frustrations in relationships originate from the evolutionary differences between the sexes. As mentioned, hormones affect emotions, which in turn motivate behaviour, so the differences in male and female hormones result in different ranges of emotions and behaviour. Hormones can affect communication styles, thinking patterns, urges and desires, methods of relaxation and ways of dealing with stress. What are these hormones, which are different on average in the male compared to the female, and how do they affect our behaviour?

First, a place of honour is given to the sex hormones, oestrogen and testosterone. As we've already seen, women and men produce both, but testosterone levels can reach 15 to 100 times higher in men than in women. Oestrogen levels vary between women and throughout the menstrual cycle, peaking during ovulation. These two hormones affect every stage of our development, from the womb to old age. They cause noticeable differences in appearance between men and women, in the face and body. These hormones are actually transcription factors: they change the expression of genes in cells and tissues. No fewer than 6,500 genes, a third of the human genome, are expressed in a man's tissue differently than in a woman's tissue (skin tissue, muscle, fat, nerve cells, liver, heart, etc.), thanks to the work of sex hormones on the genome. At week eight of pregnancy, they determine whether we will be male or female; that is, whether we will have a female or male reproductive system. Up to week eight, we are all female, which is nature's default (and, guys, if you don't believe me, the next time you look at your penis and testicles, pay attention to the prominent strip that runs between the testicles and the penis: this is a remnant of the vagina you had before week eight). At week 13, the sex hormones affect our sexual and gender orientation in the brain, dictating whether we perceive ourselves as boys or girls and to whom we will be attracted. Researchers hypothesize that the gap of five weeks in the womb, between the decision on the reproductive system and the establishment of the sexual and gender orientation in the brain, is probably the source of the wide variety of human sexual and gender orientations, which are completely natural and biological and influenced by the epigenetic effects of the womb environment.

The next step for the flow of sex hormones to the body and brain occurs at birth, and the last one is puberty; from then on it will only fluctuate over the years. During puberty, we see the effect of the sex hormones, the transcription factors, on all the tissues in the body, chest, face, waist, hips, skin, muscles, genitals, the way we smell, and all the secondary sex signs. These hormones, of course, also affect the brain, creating the sex drive and our desire to compete with members of our own gender, especially when it comes to competing for the hearts of members of the opposite sex.

Just as the sex hormones shape the body tissues of the male and female differently, so they also affect the different expressions of hormones and neurochemicals that impact our nervous system, emotions and ways of thinking and behaviour.

In chapter 4, we saw how oestrogen increases levels of oxytocin, the love hormone. The level of oxytocin in women is therefore on average two to three times higher than in men. Testosterone, on the other hand, increases the production of adrenaline and inhibits the production of oxytocin and cortisol, which means it increases the need for excitement and reduces risk aversion and empathy. Studies on risk-taking tendencies among women and men in all cultures, and also on the risk-taking of females and males in the animal kingdom, show unequivocally that females take fewer risks than males. Males are more prone to war and excitement during their lives and take bigger risks than females. Conversely, women show more empathy, the ability to recognize emotions and stronger verbal/communicative skills than men. According to data, men speak 7,000 words per day on average and women speak 21,000. These differences are due to the high level of oxytocin in women, encouraged by oestrogen, and the effect of testosterone on the male brain. At the age of 14, testosterone washes over a young boy's brain, causing a delay in the development of the communication and empathy centres and an enlargement of the amygdala gland, which is linked to stress, aggression and sex drive and is completely covered with testosterone receptors. These findings help explain why the vast majority of the most cruel acts in the world against children, women and animals have always been carried out by men. While this can be partly explained by the influence of education and society, it is also down to the biology we are born with – genes, hormones and neurons – which has a fundamental role in shaping our behaviour.

The reason for these differences is, of course, evolutionary. As noted, the reproductive strategies of males and females in nature differ. The female chooses and the male scatters. Since females can be certain their genes will be passed on to the next generation, and since they are usually the ones who bear the entire burden of raising the offspring, their reproductive strategy is to choose the male with the best genes around, the alpha, and to avoid the inferior ones. Female mice forced to mate with males they did not choose neglected their offspring. The female machine is designed for nurturing; it must therefore be focused on the needs of the offspring, show empathy, communicate, and be very careful not to take unnecessary risks.

On the other hand, for males, if he's not a winner he pretty much doesn't exist, so evolution has made him a war machine: *be ready, don't shy away from risk, take advantage of opportunities, don't show weakness, value yourself, eliminate competitors and be tough — otherwise, who will want you?* This is testosterone talking.

Perhaps it's no longer politically correct for us to speak in terms of such biological determinism. But in terms of evolution, not enough time has passed to determine whether the designs of the female nurturing machine and the male war machine no longer provide a survival advantage. In fact, the opposite appears to be true. The blurring of these designs by humans, when women refuse to nurture and men refuse to go to war, has been proven — at least from the point of view of our genes and evolution — to offer no survival advantage. This is because the end result, the only one relevant for the genes, is that those who refuse multiply less.

Whether we accept them or not, hormonal differences may surface every time we communicate as a couple, so it is important to get to know them, understand them and develop more empathy for our partner. Let's start with behavioural differences related to stress . . .

In the past, the stress response was always called "fight or flight" (no doubt because the scientists were men gathering data from males). When placed under pressure, males release more testosterone and adrenaline into the blood, which encourages the "fight and flight" response in the amygdala. On the other hand, females under stress secrete more oestrogen and oxytocin, which favour a different reaction: "freeze or tend and befriend"; in other words, freeze in place, remaining paralysed until the danger passes, or befriend someone who will take care of the offspring and help deal with the distress.

These two very different responses to stress are mediated by different hormones and are based in evolutionary logic. This is because most of the stress in females in nature is caused by males, and females with their lower muscle mass stand little chance in a fight against men or in running away from them – and, anyway, what about the children? Such a response is doomed to failure. That's why evolution has favoured females who respond in a way that is more suitable to their core attributes – by freezing in place, waiting for it to be over and being left alone again. The freezing response can also explain the common and infuriating question that often arises in relation to sexual assaults and harassment: *Why didn't you run away? Why didn't you shout?* The fact is that the body enters a state of system shutdown. The second response is to take care of your offspring, call friends who will help you process the trauma, be nice to everyone and move on. A brief look at human history shows what happened to those women who dared to fight, resist and run away, compared to women who suffered in silence, protected their offspring and vented their frustration with friends.

The effects of these hormones also play out in marital quarrels. All of us, women and men alike, fight, run away, freeze in place or seek consolation with someone. However, on average men are more likely to run away from a confrontation or an outburst of rage when they can't stand it anymore, whereas women will stay in a verbal exchange that can be aggressive, critical, even venomous. Women freeze on the spot in the face of another's outburst and may then rehash the quarrel in conversations with their social circle.

In addition to oxytocin, which promotes post-event rumination, the base level of cortisol in a woman's blood is two to three times higher than in men. As mentioned, testosterone is responsible for reducing cortisol secretion in males. During an argument, this leads to women needing on average twice as long to calm down as men. Cortisol remains in the blood for between 20 and 40 minutes.

Worldwide data show that women suffer two to three times more anxiety and depression than men. In fact, the population group that has the highest risk of clinical depression is mothers with young children. Their high cortisol levels cause women to suffer ten times more from eating disorders than men, and to be significantly more prone to autoimmune diseases after the age of 40. These are diseases in which the immune system goes out of control and attacks the body, following the harmful effect of cortisol as it suppresses the immune system. Common post-traumatic symptoms in women can manifest differently than in men. They will appear as emotional numbness, avoidance, mood swings, anxiety and depression disorders, shame and self-blame. In men, they may present themselves as impatience and irritability, tantrums, impulsiveness, escape into addictive substances, paranoia, wariness and hypervigilance.

During quarrels and more generally during times of stress, women are more likely to cry. Why is this? In the Department of Neurobiology at Israel's Weizmann Institute of Science, a fascinating study was carried out a few years ago in the laboratory of Professor Noam Sobel. A curious poster was displayed around the research institute: "We want people who cry in movies and commercials." Several women and one man accepted the invitation.

During the experiment, the subjects were asked to watch sad movies and collect their tears in a test tube. The researchers then had other people smell the women's tears and also a saline solution, which was used as a control sample. Amazingly, the genuine tears caused the testosterone level in the men's blood to drop by 20 per cent within half an hour! We know of no other external stimulus that affects the level of hormones in the blood like that. It turns out that our tears contain pheromones, those volatile derivatives of the sex hormones, which pass through the olfactory epithelium to the brain of the person smelling them – and cause a decrease in testosterone in the blood. Crying is not a weakness, it is an evolutionary superpower for lowering testosterone, damping down the aggression of those who try to hurt us. This is why babies cry all the time, because in the wild when they are born they are exposed to the deadly aggression of males toward their cubs. The next time tears appear in a quarrel, remember the pheromones in those tears and their purpose.

Statistics show that most crises between spouses develop about three years after the birth of their first child. Psychologists and relationship therapists describe a variety of ways in which raising children disrupts marital harmony. However, our primary concern here is in the role of biology. As we have seen, during pregnancy and childbirth, a woman's body and mind undergo significant changes. The brain is subjected to a fundamental reorganization, with an increase in the number of oxytocin-releasing neurons in the pleasure system and structural changes in the white matter and grey matter of the brain. This is for the benefit of strengthening pathways in the nurturing, empathy and communication areas of the brain at the expense of other pathways.

Researchers from the University of Barcelona in Spain carried out MRI examinations of the brains of 25 women before and after their first pregnancy and compared these to the brains of women who did not become pregnant, and to men's brains. The researchers discovered a significant reduction in grey matter in the brains of the pregnant women, which was concentrated in the same areas of the brain in all these women. The reduction was so great that, based on the change in grey matter volume, the researchers could determine whether a particular woman was pregnant or not.

The grey matter in the brain consists of the bodies of the nerve cells, while the white matter comprises the long fibres of the nerve cells, which make connections between neurons and with the sensory and motor systems. The reduction in the volume of the grey matter probably indicates the processes of specialization the brain undergoes. The last time a pregnant woman's brain underwent a comparable amount of change in the grey matter was during puberty. During this period, the human brain experiences changes in the synapses (connections) between the brain cells, in a process called "neural pruning". These changes are essential to our emotional and cognitive development as teenagers. During pregnancy, a similar process takes place in certain areas of the woman's brain that have been found to be linked to social behaviour, empathic abilities and interpersonal relationships. The researchers from Barcelona hypothesized that the purpose of these changes is to make the brain more efficient with respect to the woman developing mothering skills, establishing an emotional connection with the baby and being alert and oriented to its needs. Making her a nurturing machine, as we said.

Indeed, when the researchers watched the activity in the mothers' brains while they were shown pictures of their babies, they saw increased activity in the same areas where the grey matter had been reduced. A positive relationship was also found between the changes in the brain and the extent of the women's attachment to their babies, as assessed by their responses to questionnaires.

The trigger for all these events in a mother's mind are the hormones that flood her body during pregnancy, the placental hormone, progesterone, oestrogen (which encourages the secretion of oxytocin and prolactin), adrenaline and cortisol. These hormones affect all the tissues, systems and organs of the body. They effect changes in metabolism, bodily fluids, the energy system, the digestive tract, the excretory system, the blood system, the immune system, the management of fat reserves, the development of the breasts and much more. In addition, these hormones also greatly affect a woman's emotional and mental health.

Oestrogen and progesterone bring about changes in self-image, with oestrogen causing pleasant and uplifting feelings, while progesterone lowers self-confidence. Rapid changes in these hormones also bring sharp mood changes, and after birth, when they plummet, women are at risk of getting the "baby blues", feeling down and even depressed.

Oxytocin produces the feeling of connection to the baby, the desire to connect with people, reconcile with parents, seek out community and prepare a social network for the mother and baby.

Prolactin encourages breast development during pregnancy. After birth, the level of it increases and encourages the production of milk. The prolactin level remains high in breastfeeding mothers and, together with oxytocin, strengthens the emotional attachment between mother and newborn. Prolactin also suppresses ovulation and the new mother's libido. After all, from a biological perspective, the "nurturing machine" shouldn't be interested in attracting males at the moment; it only needs to be focused on taking care of the baby. Prolactin is the hormone secreted in men and women immediately after orgasm that triggers the delay mechanism, making it impossible to reach another orgasm immediately. Prolactin lowers the levels of testosterone and oestrogen and with them the sex drive.

And if prolactin, which destroys happiness, is not bad enough, we women have oestrogen and progesterone messing with our mood and self-image, and finally cortisol and adrenaline, the stress hormones. Stress hormones are secreted mostly during the last trimester of pregnancy, so that the "nurturing machine" is alert and ready to protect itself and its baby, which is about to emerge into a dangerous world. Cortisol is already at work erasing any sexual desire that might surface in the new mother.

And what happens to the father all this time? He doesn't go through pregnancy, he doesn't experience childbirth and there is no massive reorganization event in his mind. Ninety-five per cent of females in nature take care of their offspring without assistance from their fathers and dedicate most of their lives and bodies to this work. In humans, unlike other male mammals, fathers increasingly fill a role in child care. Due to this, these fathers also go through certain hormonal changes as they spend time together with the mother and/or the baby. The level of testosterone in the man's blood decreases when he is with them, his oxytocin rises and his cortisol levels climb to match closely those of the mother. This is all thanks to the mirror neurons. The father might experience mood changes, stress and also a strong connection to his partner and the baby. However, since the changes in the new father occur more slowly and not with the same intensity as in the mother, he may often feel confused, abandoned and out of place in the household. The relationship between a father and his children is formed over time, through the joint creation of oxytocin via contact, play, talking and shared quality time.

These differences in the changes in the mind and body of the new mother compared to those experienced by the father explain a lot of the conflicts that come to the surface when two become three.

The oxytocin and the changes in her brain's empathy and communication centres cause her to tune in to every chirp, cry or purr. The mirror neuron activity in her brain moves into high gear, and she will sense her baby's needs in ways that sometimes seem telepathic. Studies have shown that mothers have an incredible ability to recognize their baby's cries among the wails of other babies. The father, on the other hand, will not always immediately recognize his baby's needs, nor will he necessarily be able to be equally attentive to every nuance of the baby's cries. As a result of this difference, conflicts, disagreements and quarrels may develop between the couple regarding the children's needs and their upbringing, all of which will accompany them long after the children grow up.

On top of that, the hormonal swing of pregnancy, childbirth and raising small children can widen the gaps in the couple's sex drive. To begin with, the basic data is not promising, with 15 to 100 times more testosterone in the man, a reproductive system that produces an average of five times greater sex drive and thinking about sex a lot more often. After the birth of the baby, there is no significant damage to the man's sex drive. On the contrary, the increase in oxytocin in the new father and the strong sense of connection to his partner, the mother of his children, will actually create sexual arousal and increase his desire to connect with her through intimacy and intercourse. This is to proportional to the extent that the man doesn't experience, together with his partner, an increase in cortisol, following postpartum depression. Mum's sex drive, however, has never been lower, due to the variety of desire-suppressing and nurture-stimulating hormones, coupled with a lack of sleep, worries, multitasking, and constant fatigue. This is where the slippery slope of self-blame, partner blame, mutual frustration, shame and accumulated resentment begins. All of these may lead to an increase in the number of unnecessary quarrels over small and insignificant matters, because no one is talking about the elephant in the room – *what has happened to our sex life since the children arrived?*

If we revisit the example of the female orangutan in the wild, we saw how she retires after the birth of her young and isolates herself to raise it in peace. She isn't interested in males at all. Only after eight years, when the "chick has flown the nest", will the level of oestrogen in her blood recover. Then, she will feel sexually motivated and resolutely go after the alpha male on duty in the vicinity. She will go on a three-day whirlwind honeymoon with him, get pregnant and retire again to raise her new offspring.

Understanding how the different biology and chemistry of the female and male body and brain shape our behaviour, ways of coping and thinking, can help us build a relationship that better supports our different abilities and needs. Ignoring and denying the biological differences that evolution has instilled in us for millions of years, for the purpose of survival, can harm the relationships of both women and men. Gender empathy in a relationship – recognizing the differences between us as men and women – lets us step into our partner's shoes; to understand consciously that what we are going through, they are not necessarily going through; what we feel, they do not always feel. The way we deal with difficulty is not necessarily going to be our partner's strategy, and the way we ask for love is not necessarily the way they ask for love. The solution is, as always, empathy.

CONCLUSION

More than a decade ago, I embarked on a fascinating journey to explore the story of love. The loves I experienced, the disappointments I inherited and the choices I took, made me want to truly understand the basis of my behaviour when it comes to love, the way I make my decisions and the impulses and emotions that drive me. As a scientist who looks at the world through the lens of biology and evolution, I equipped myself with all the tools that the world of science has made available to me and set out to investigate the neurons, hormones and genes that shape our love lives. Although a selfish instinct encouraged me to think that I was special in some way, a quick look around showed me that when it comes to love, I certainly don't behave differently from the rest of my friends and fellow humans.

In these pages, it has been my pleasure to share the knowledge I have gathered with you, with the aim of helping us all get to know ourselves more deeply and use this knowledge to improve our relationships with our partners.

I have often been asked, "In the end, doesn't all this knowledge damage my love life? Does the knowledge that everything is a product of brain chemistry and that our genes actually manage us behind the scenes harm my ability to find love?"

I say the opposite is true. As I mentioned at the very start of this book, I believe that to understand something is to be freed from it. When we understand the motivations for our emotions and behaviour and we operate from the conscious parts of the brain – rather than the unconscious, automatic parts – we can control our behaviour. Many of our disappointments, certainly when it comes to love, stem from irrational and instinctive behaviour dictated by evolutionary codes and algorithms. Once we become aware of these codes and instincts and understand them, we can control them – instead of allowing them to control us.

We are not chimpanzees, monkeys or mice; we have a prefrontal lobe. This is the conscious, thinking, rational third of the brain, which has evolved since we separated from the chimpanzees five million years ago. It is this part that enables us to have an intellectual discussion today about the biology and chemistry of our love lives, to analyse our instincts and urges, in a way that is not possible for any other animal on Earth.

Today, for the first time in human history, each and every one of us has both the knowledge and the freedom to choose what will be good for us. Today, women and men, at least in the Western world, are allowed to choose the best love life for them; to get married at whatever age they want, or not get married; to have children in whatever family configuration suits them, or not have children at all.

As we have seen, this freedom involves limitations and disadvantages. The multitude of choices in the digital dating world causes cognitive flooding and we become overcritical. The way that the biological clock ticks differently in men and women can cause frustration, since the promise that 30 is the new 20 holds no validity for women, as the uterus hasn't changed for thousands of years and a woman's fertility still drops significantly from age 33. Furthermore, in the age of plenty in which we are living in the developed world – with an abundance of resources and an abundance of temptations – there is no evolutionary advantage in lifelong monogamy. Where there is abundance, our genes push for diversification and spreading risk. And so in an age of single people swamped with technology, it is even more important to understand the science of love, what lies behind our choices, how to choose correctly and how to sustain love over time.

On a personal level, I have no doubt that if, at the age of 20, I had been equipped with the knowledge I have acquired about love now that I've reached 45, it is very possible that my love life would have looked different. I probably wouldn't have married my first boyfriend, whom I met at the age of 18. I would have accepted that my teenage mind was flooded with powerful love drugs for the first time in my life, rendering me unable to see all the parameters essential for making an informed decision like a wedding. In a situation where the prefrontal lobe is still maturing and the emotional brain is flooded, splitting up was only a matter of time; in my case, two and a half years.

One can assume that I would have been more wary of toxic relationships, too, had I the knowledge to spot the signs of a toxic relationship and recognize people who are incapable of love.

It is also possible that I would not have rushed to marry a second time at the age of 28, due to the strong attraction I felt for a stranger. During a trip to faraway Nepal, when I was fascinated by the landscapes and people, flooded with dopamine and adrenaline, I fell in love with the most attractive Nepali guy. In my case, an adrenaline rush experienced during a trip (which happens to virtually every young man and woman) ended once again in a wedding. If I had known that we have a biological evolutionary tendency to be attracted to the different and unfamiliar – but for psychological reasons, the familiar attractions are those that endure – I might have postponed the wedding.

And perhaps my conduct in a later relationship might have been different if, for example, I had known, after giving birth, about the destructive effect of prolactin on the life of a couple raising small children. Things would have been different if I had understood in detail what was happening to my brain and body during pregnancy and birth, and how evolution turned me into a nurturing machine, someone focused on maternal anxiety and a less sexual being. A deadly trinity for a relationship to face.

I do not regret any decision I have made in my life. I have learned from every experience I've had, and I have also had the privilege of bringing into the world the most precious creatures to me, my oxytocin creatures, my beloved children Maya and Milan.

At the age of 41, when my frontal lobe fully matured and my emotional brain knew how to regulate itself better, I was able for the third (and last) time to choose a partner who suits me, and finally manage my love life with full awareness. I found calm and comfort in the familiar. My partner, Erez, with his kindness, his charm, his marital and familial nature and even his appearance evoked strong oxytocin memories in me from my past, memories of the significant caring figure in my life, my blessed father, who took care of me and my siblings with endless devotion and taught me everything I know about love.

"All you need is love," the Beatles sang long ago. Indeed, we were born for love, born for oxytocin. Our brain needs the love hormone to develop and thrive from our time in the womb and into old age. Like many other mammals, we humans are sociable creatures who are completely dependent on each other for our survival. Loneliness is bad for us. Our nervous system needs the proximity of another nervous system to relax. We relax when we are in the company of people, it is an integral part of our biology. In an age that has very recently experienced epidemics and social distancing, we need to understand, more than ever, the consequences of these actions on our emotional and mental health. We are wired for love, for social connection, and we find meaning in helping the people dear to us and promoting the wellbeing of our human sisters and brothers. This is what makes us human.

NOTES

	Page	Paragraph
The Emotional Brain: The Mysterious Underpinnings of Emotional Life, Joseph Ledoux, Simon & Schuster 1998	2	
G. Rizzolatti, L. Fadiga, V. Gallese ı L. Fogassi, "Premotor cortex and the recognition of motor actions," Cognitive Brain Research ,3 ,pp. 131-141, 1996 .	4	3
G. Rizzolatti ı S. Corrado, Mirrors in the Brain: How Our Minds Share Actions, Emotions, and Experience, Oxford University Press, 2008 .	4	3
P. J. Zack, The Moral Molecule: The Source of Love and Prosperity, Dutton, 2012 .	5	2
P. J. Zack, The Moral Molecule: The Source of Love and Prosperity, Dutton, 2012 .	5, 53	2, 1
Carter CS, Porges SW. The biochemistry of love: an oxytocin hypothesis. EMBO Rep. 2013 Jan;14(1):12-6. doi: 10.1038/embor.2012.191. Epub 2012 Nov 27.	6	
S. W. Porges, The Polyvagal Theory: Neurophysiological Foundations of Emotions, Attachment, Communication, and Self-Regulation, Barnes and Noble, 2011 .	6	
E. Madsen, R. Tunney, G. Fieldman, H. Plotkin, R. Dunbar, J.-M. Richardson ı D. McFarland, "Kinship and altruism: A cross-cultural experimental study," British Journal of Psychology ,98 ,p. 339–359, 2007 .	7	3
C. Darwin, The Descent of Man, and Selection in Relation to Sex, London .	8	2
H. Eiberg, J. Troelsen, M. Nielsen, A. Mikkelsen, J. Mengel-From, K. W. Kjaer ı L. Hansen, "Blue eye color in humans may be caused by a perfectly associated founder mutation in a regulatory element located within the HERC2 gene inhibiting OCA2 expression," Human Genetics ,123 ,p. 177–187, 2008.	9	2
K. Schmida, M. David ı A. Samalc, "Computation of a face attractiveness index based on neoclassical canons, symmetry, and golden ratios," Pattern Recognition ,8 ,41 ,pp. 2710-2717, 2008 .	10	3
S. Richmond, L. Howe, S. Lewis, S. Evie ı A. Zhurov, "Facial Genetics: A Brief Overview," Frontiers in Genetics, 2018 .	10	4
S. Geniole, T. Denson, B. Dixson, J. Carré ı C. McCormick, "Evidence from Meta-Analyses of the Facial Width-to-Height Ratio as an Evolved Cue of Threat," Plos One ,7 ,10 ,p. e0132726, 2015 .	11	3
M. J. Law-Smith, D. I. Perrett, B. C. Jones, R. E. Cornwell, F. R. Moore, D. R. Feinberg, L. G. Boothroyd, S. J. Durrani, M. R. Stirrat, S. Whiten, R. M. Pitman ı H. S. G, "Facial appearance is a cue to oestrogen levels in women," Proceedings of the Royal Society B: Biological Sciences ,1583 ,273 ,p. 135–140, 2006 .	11	4
E. Bruch, F. Feinberg ı K. Y. Lee, "Extracting multistage screening rules from online dating activity data," Proceedings of the National Academy of Sciences ,38 ,113 ,pp. 10530-10535, August 2016 .	12	1
J. Shepperd ı A. Strathman, "Attractiveness and Height: The Role of Stature in Dating Preference, Frequency of Dating, and Perceptions of Attractiveness," Personality and Social Psychology Bulletin, 1989 .	12	2
J. Pinsker, "The Financial Perks of Being Tall," The Atlantic, 2015.	12	2
N. Li, J. Yong, W. Tov, O. Sng, G. Fletcher, K. Valentine, Y. Jiang ı D. Balliet, "Mate preferences do predict attraction and choices in the early stages of mate selection," Journal of Personality and Social Psychology ,5 ,105 ,pp. 757-76, 2013 .	12	3
L. Waterlow, "Size matters in online dating: Short men get less interest from women than their taller counterparts - and those at 6ft have the most luck," 2013[on-line] dailymail.co.uk	12	1
S. Walters ı C. Crawford, "The importance of mate attraction for intrasexual competition in men and women," Ethology and Sociobiology ,1 ,15 ,pp. 5-30, 1994 .	13	2
A. Aron, E. Melinat, E. Aron, R. Vallone ı B. Renee, "The Experimental Generation of Interpersonal Closeness: A Procedure and Some Preliminary Findings," Personality and Social Psychology Bulletin, 1997 .	14	2
John G. H. Cant. "Hypothesis for the Evolution of Human Breasts and Buttocks." The American Naturalist, vol. 117, no. 2, 1981, pp. 199–204. JSTOR, www.jstor.org/stable/2460501. Accessed 23 Sept. 2023.	15	
S. Tifferet, O. Gaziel ı Y. Baram, "Guitar Increases Male Facebook Attractiveness: Preliminary Support for the Sexual Selection Theory of Music," Letters of Evolutionary Behavioral Science ,1 ,3 ,pp. 4-6, 2012 .	16	2
A. Zahavi ı A. Zahavi, The Handicap Principle: A Missing Piece of Darwin's Puzzle, Oxford University Press, 1997 .	16	3
S. Street, T. Morgan, A. Thornton, G. Brown, K. Laland ı C. Cross, "Human mate-choice copying is domain-general social learning," Scientific Reports .2018 ,1 ,8 ,	17	3
C. Wedekind, T. Seebeck, F. Bettens ı A. Paepke, "MHC-dependent mate preferences in humans," Proceedings of the Royal Society of London. Series B: Biological Sciences .1995 ,1359 ,260 ,	18	2
S. Kirshenbaum, The Science of Kissing: What Our Lips Are Telling Us, Grand Central Publishing, 2011 .	19	2

C. Wyart, W. Webster, J. Chen, S. Wilson, A. McClary, R. Khan ı N. Sobel, "Smelling a Single Component of Male Sweat Alters Levels of Cortisol in Women," Journal of Neuroscience ,6 ,27 ,pp. 1261-1265, 2007 .	19	3
T. Saxton, A. Lyndon, A. Little ı C. Roberts, "Evidence that androstadienone, a putative human chemosignal, modulates women's attributions of men's attractiveness," Hormones and Behavior ,54 , ,5pp. 597-601, 2008 .	19	3
M. J. Olsson, J. N. Lundström, S. Diamantopoulou ı F. Estevesa, "A putative female pheromone affects mood in men differently depending on social context," European Review of Applied Psychology ,56 , ,4pp. 279-284, 2006 .	19	3
CNN, "Sniff out your soul mate at a pheromone party – creator Judith Prays explains how it works," CNN, 2012.	20	1
Westermarck, Edvard A. (1921). The History of Human Marriage (5th ed.). London: Macmillan	20	last
Incest. A biosocial view. By J. Shepher. New York: Academic Press. 1983. xiv 213 pp	21	1
Wolf, Arthur P. (2005). "Chapter 4: Explaining the Westermarck effect, or, what did natural selection select for?". In Wolf, Arthur P.; Durham, William H. (eds.). Inbreeding, Incest, and the Incest Taboo: The State of Knowledge at the Turn of the Century. Stanford, California: Stanford University Press.	21	3
Malikov, Azim. (2018). Kinship Systems of Xoja Groups in Southern Kazakhstan. Anthropology of the Middle East. 12. 10.3167/ame.2017.120206.	22	1
https://www.ethiopianorthodox.org/biography/02thelawofkings.pdf	22	1
B. Laeng, O. Vermeer ı S. Unni, "Is Beauty in the Face of the Beholder?" Plos One, 2013 .	23	1
M. Robinson, A. Kleinman, M. Graff, A. Vinkhuyzen, D. Couper, M. Miller, W. Peyrot, A. Abdellaoui, B. Zietsch, I. Nolte, J. v. Vliet-Ostaptchouk ı H. Snieder, "Genetic evidence of assortative mating in humans," Nature Human Behaviour ,1 ,p. 16, 2017 .	23	3
T. Bereczkei, G. Petra ı G. Weisfeld, "Sexual imprinting in human mate choice," Proceedings of the Royal Society B: Biological Sciences ,271 ,pp. 1129-1134, 2004 .	24	1
M. Vicedo, "The Father of Ethology and the Foster Mother of Ducks: Konrad Lorenz as Expert on Motherhood," University of Chicago Press .2009 ,2 'בn ,100 ,	24	2
I. P. Owens, C. Rowe ı T. A. L, "Sexual selection, speciation and imprinting: separating the sheep from the goats ."	24	3
T. Bereczkei, P. Gyuris, P. Koves ı L. Bernath, "Homogamy, genetic similarity, and imprinting; parental influence on mate choice preferences," Personality and Individual Differences ,5 ,33 ,pp. 677-690, 2002 .	25	2
C. Roberts, M. Gosling, V. Carter ı M. Petrie, "MHC-correlated odour preferences in humans and the use of oral contraceptives," Proceedings of the Royal Society B: Biological Sciences ,1652 ,275 ,pp. 2715-22, 2008 .	26	6
Roberts, S. C., Little, A. C., Burriss, R. P., Cobey, K. D., Klapilová, K., Havlíček, J., Jones, B. C., DeBruine, L., & Petrie, M. (2014). Partner Choice, Relationship Satisfaction, and Oral Contraception: The Congruency Hypothesis. Psychological Science, 25(7), 1497–1503.	26	5
Geoffrey Miller, Joshua M. Tybur, Brent D. Jordan, Ovulatory cycle effects on tip earnings by lap dancers: economic evidence for human estrus? Evolution and Human Behavior, Volume 28, Issue 6, 2007, Pages 375-381,	27	2
Sexual side effects of SSRIs: Why it happens and what to do Coping with this common side effect from antidepressants.	27	last
July 7, 2023, Reviewed by Howard E. LeWine, MD, Chief Medical Editor, Harvard Health Publishing Fisher, HE and JA Thomson (2007) Lust, Attraction, Attachment: Do the side effects of serotoninenhancing antidepressants jeopardize romantic love, marriage and fertility? In S Platek, JP Keenan and TK Shackelford (Eds.) Evolutionary Cognitive Neuroscience. Cambridge, MA: MIT Press. Pp 245-283	28	1
H. Fisher, Why We Love: The Nature and Chemistry of Romantic Love, Holt Paperbacks, 2004 .	28	1
P. Backus, "Why I don't have a girlfriend - an application of the Drake equation to love in the UK," 1999.	29	2
J. Kincaid, "OkCupid Checks Out the Dynamics of Attraction And Your Love Inbox," Techcrunch, 2009 . [on-line] techcrunch.com/2009	29	1
E-harmony, "One in 562 - the odds of finding love," 2009 [on-line] thirdcity.co.uk	29	2
B. Shivali, "Mathematicians reveal odds finding love," August 2017 .[on-line] dailymail.co.uk.	29	4
H. Fry, The Mathematics of Love: Patterns, Proofs and the Search for the Ultimate Equation, Ted Books, 2015 .	30	1
M. Freiberger, "Strategic dating: The 37% rule," Plus Magazine .	31	3
Plus Magazine, "Kissing the frog: A mathematician's guide to mating," Plus Magazine .	31	3
M. Iqbal, "Tinder Revenue and Usage Statistics (2021)," 2021.	32	last
VIDA Select, "Should I Lie in My Online Dating Profile."	33	2
S. Rosenbloom, "Love, Lies and What They Learned," The New York Times, pp. Section ST, Page 1, November 2011.	33	2

		33	2

R. Epstein, "The Truth about Online Dating," Scientific American Mind, 3, 20, 54-61, 2009 . — 33 — 2

B. Schwartz, The Paradox of Choice - Why More is Less. How The Culture of Abundance Robs Us of Satisfaction, Harper Perennial, 2004 . — 34 — 2

Hate It or Love It, Tinder's Right Swipe Limit Is Working Jordan Crook, techcrunch.com — 35 — 3

C. B. Ferster ۱ B. F. Skinner, Schedules of reinforcement, Appleton-Century-Crofts, 1957 . — 35 — last

B. F. Skinner, Science and human behavior, New York: The Free Press, 1953 . — 36 — 3

A. Paul, "Is Online Better Than Offline for Meeting Partners? Depends: Are You Looking to Marry or to Date?," Cyberpsychology, Behavior, and Social Networking. 2014, 10, 17 — 37 — 1

Traister, Rebecca. All the Single Ladies: Unmarried Women and the Rise of an Independent Nation Simon & Schuster, 2016 — 39 — 3

B. Rammstedta, F. Spinath, D. Richter ۱ J. Schupp, "Partnership longevity and personality congruence in couples," Personality and Individual Differences, 7, 54, 832-835, 2013 . — 40 — 3

Wikipedia, "List of animals displaying homosexual behavior. — 42 — 2

H. Osborne, "More Gay Dolphins Observed Off Coast of Western Australia," 2017 [on-line] ,newsweek.com — 42 — 2

A. Barron ۱ B. Hare, "Prosociality and a Sociosexual Hypothesis for the Evolution of Same-Sex Attraction in Humans," Frontiers in Psychology, 2020 . — 43 — 1

J. Barthesa, B. Godellea ۱ M. Raymondb, "Human social stratification and hypergyny: toward an understanding of male homosexual preference," Evolution and Human Behaviour, 3, 34, 155-163, 2013 . — 43 — 4

D. Hamer, S. Hu, V. Magnuson, N. Hu ۱ A. Pttatucci, "A linkage between DNA markers on the X chromosome and male sexual orientation," Science, 5119, 261, כרך , 321-7, 1993 . — 44 — 2

A. Sanders, G. Beecham, S. Guo, K. Dawood, G. Rieger, J. Badner, E. Gershon, R. Krishnappa, A. Kolundzija, J. Duan, P. Gejman, M. Bailey ۱ E. Martin, "Genome-Wide Association Study of Male Sexual Orientation," Nature, p. 16950, 2017 . — 44 — 3

A. Ganna, K. Verweij, M. Nivard, R. Maier, R. Wedow, A. Busch, A. Abdellaoui, S. Guo, J. F. Sathirapongsasuti, 2. Team Research ۱ P. Lichtenstein, "Large-scale GWAS reveals insights into the genetic architecture of same-sex sexual behavior," Science, 6456, 365, 7693, 2019 . — 44 — 4

J. Balthazart, "Fraternal birth order effect on sexual orientation explained," Proceedings of the National Academy of Sciences, 2, 115, 234–236, 2018 . — 45 — 2

A. F. Bogaert, M. Skorska, C. Wang, J. Gabrie, A. MacNeil, M. Hoffarth, D. VanderLaan, K. Zucker ۱ R. Blanchard, "Male homosexuality and maternal immune responsivity to the Y-linked protein NLGN4Y," Proceedings of the National Academy of Sciences, 2, 115, 302-306, 2018 . — 45 — 3

S. Nila, P.-A. Crochet, J. Barthes, P. Rianti, B. Juliandi, B. Suryobroto ۱ M. Raymond, "Male Homosexual Preference: Femininity and the Older Brother Effect in Indonesia," Evolutionary Psychology, 4, 17 . 2019 . — 45 — 4

A. F. Bogaert ۱ M. Skorska, "Sexual orientation, fraternal birth order, and the maternal immune hypothesis: a review," Frontiers in Neuroendocrinology, 2, 32, 247-54, 2011 . — 45 — 5

Bogaert AF, Skorska MN, Wang C, Gabrie J, MacNeil AJ, Hoffarth MR, VanderLaan DP, Zucker KJ, Blanchard R. Male homosexuality and maternal immune responsivity to the Y-linked protein NLGN4Y. Proc Natl Acad Sci U S A. 2018 Jan 9;115(2):302-306. doi: 10.1073/pnas.1705895114. Epub 2017 Dec — 46 — 2

F. Galis, C. Ten Broek, S. Van Dongen ۱ L. Wijnaendts, "Sexual Dimorphism in the Prenatal Digit Ratio (2D:4D)," Archives of Sexual Behavior, 1, 39, 57–62, 2010 . — 47 — 2

B. Gladue, W. Beatty, J. Larson ۱ D. Staton, "Sexual orientation and spatial ability in men and women," Psychobiology, 18, 101-8, 1990 . — 47 — 3

E. Hampson ۱ S. Janani, "Hand preference in humans is associated with testosterone levels and androgen receptor gene polymorphism," Neuropsychologia, 8, 50, 2018-25, 2012 . — 47 — 4

W. Rice, U. Friberg ۱ S. Gavrilets, "Homosexuality as a Consequence of Epigenetically Canalized Sexual Development," The Quarterly Review of Biology, 4, 87, 343-368, 2012 . — 48 — 2

T. Ngun ۱ E. Vilain, "The biological basis of human sexual orientation: is there a role for epigenetics?" Advances in Genetics, 86, 167-184, 2014 . — 48 — last

Kinsey, Alfred C., Wardell B. Pomeroy, and Clyde E. Martin. Sexual Behavior in the Human Male. Philadelphia, PA: W. B. Saunders Company, 1948 — 49 — last

Attanasio M, Masedu F, Quattrini F, Pino MC, Vagnetti R, Valenti M, Mazza M. Are Autism Spectrum Disorder and Asexuality Connected? Arch Sex Behav. 2022 May;51(4):2091-2115. — 50 — 1

Baettig L, Baeumelt A, Ernst J, Boeker H, Grimm S, Richter A. The awareness of the scared - context dependent influence of oxytocin on brain function. Brain Imaging Behav. 2020 Dec;14(6):2073-2083 — 53 — 1

onobo Sex and Society" in SA Special Editions 16, 3s, 14-21, June 2006 — 54 — 1

Nave, Gideon, Amos Nadler, David Zava, ۱ Colin Camerer. 2017. "Single Dose Testosterone Administration Impairs Cognitive Reflection in Men". Psychological Science 28 (10): 1398–1407. — 54 — last

Serum Testosterone Levels in Sex offenders, P O Gurnani M Dwyer. Journal of Offender Counseling, Services and Rehabilitation Volume: 11 Issue: 1 Dated: (Fall -Winter 1986) Pages: 39-45 — 55 — 1

Pope HG Jr, Kouri EM, Hudson JI. Effects of supraphysiologic doses of testosterone on mood and aggression in normal men: a randomized controlled trial. Arch Gen Psychiatry. 2000 Feb;57(2):133-40; discussion 155-6.   55   1

Sprouse-Blum AS, Smith G, Sugai D, Parsa FD. Understanding endorphins and their importance in pain management. Hawaii Med J. 2010 Mar;69(3):70-1.   55   last

Young LJ, Flanagan-Cato LM. Editorial comment: oxytocin, vasopressin and social behavior. Horm Behav. 2012 Mar;61(3):227-9   59   1

T. H. C. Kruger, "Specificity of the neuroendocrine response to orgasm during sexual arousal in men," Journal of Endocrinology ,1 ,177 ,57-64, 2003 .   59   2

J. T. Winslow, N. Hastings, C. S. Carter, C. R. Harbaugh ı T. R. Insel, "A role for central vasopressin in pair bonding in monogamous prairie voles," Nature ,6446 ,365 , 545-8, 1993 .   59   5

Kruger, Tillmann. (2003). Specificity of the neuroendocrine response to orgasm during sexual arousal in men. Journal of Endocrinology. 177. 57-64.   59   2

P. Wang, H.-P. Yang, S. Tian, L. Wang, S. Wang, F. Zhang ı Y.-F. Wang, "Oxytocin-secreting system: A major part of the neuroendocrine center regulating immunologic activity," Journal of Neuroimmunology ,289 ,152-61, 2015 .   60   3

Gabry KE. The Science of Orgasm. JAMA. 2008;299(6):701–702.   60   last

M. Leitzmann, E. Platz, M. Stampfer, W. Willett ı E. Giovannucci, "Ejaculation frequency and subsequent risk of prostate cancer," The Journal of Urology ,13 , 291 , 1578-86, 2004 .   61   3

S. Ortigue, F. Bianchi-Demicheli, N. Patel, C. Frum ı J. Lewis, "Neuroimaging of Love: fMRI Meta-Analysis Evidence toward New Perspectives in Sexual Medicine," The Journal of Sexual Medicine ,7 , ,113541-3552, 2010 .   63   2

R. Burriss, C. Roberts, L. Welling, D. Puts ı A. Little, "Heterosexual Romantic Couples Mate Assortatively for Facial Symmetry, But Not Masculinity," Personality and Social Psychology Bulletin , ,5 ,37601-13, 2011 .   63   4

P. Bos, D. Hofman, E. Hermans, E. Montoya, S. Baron-Cohen ı J. van-Honk, "Testosterone reduces functional connectivity during the 'Reading the Mind in the Eyes' Test," Psychoneuroendocrinology , ,68194-201, 2016 .   64   3

S. Okabe, K. Kitano, M. Nagasawa, K. Mogi ı T. Kikusui, "Testosterone inhibits facilitating effects of parenting experience on parental behavior and the oxytocin neural system in mice," Physiology & Behavior ,118 ,159-164, 2013 .   64   3

E. H. Albers, "The regulation of social recognition, social communication and aggression: Vasopressin in the social behavior neural network," Hormones and Behavior ,3 ,61 ,283-292, 2012 .   65   4

Y. Delville, K. Mansour ı C. Ferris, "Testosterone facilitates aggression by modulating vasopressin receptors in the hypothalamus," Physiology & Behavior ,1 ,60 ,25-29, 1996 .   65   4

M. Mcclure, "Stanford researchers discover the African cichlid's noisy courtship ritual," Stanford Report, 2012.   65   5

J. Desjardins, J. Klausner ı R. Fernald, "Female genomic response to mate information," Proceedings of the National Academy of Sciences ,49 ,107 , 21176-21180, 2010 .   65   5

M. Shwartz, "Social status triggers genetic response in male cichlid fish," Stanford Report, 2005.   65   last

G. Doron, D. Derby ı O. Szepsenwol, "Relationship obsessive compulsive disorder (ROCD): A conceptual framework," Journal of Obsessive-Compulsive and Related Disorders ,2 ,3 ,169–180, 2014 .   68   2

C. Riley, "The dolphin who loved me: the Nasa-funded project that went wrong," The Guardian, 2014 .   70   2

CDC Vital Signs Report, June 2018   71   2

Patankar GR, Choi JW, Schussler JM. Reverse takotsubo cardiomyopathy: two case reports and review of the literature. Journal of Medical Case Reports. 2013; 7:84   71   last

J. Holt-Lunstad, T. Smith, M. Baker, T. Harris ı D. Stephenson, "Loneliness and Social Isolation as Risk Factors for Mortality: A Meta-Analytic Review," Perspectives on Psychological Science, 2015 .   72   last

Bowlby, J. (1979). The Bowlby-Ainsworth attachment theory. Behavioral and Brain Sciences, 2(4), 637-638   74   last

Servin-Barthet, C., Martínez-García, M., Pretus, C. et al. The transition to motherhood: linking hormones, brain and behaviour. Nat. Rev. Neurosci. 24, 605–619 (2023).   77   3

M. Pereira, "Structural and Functional Plasticity in the Maternal Brain Circuitry," New Directions for Child and Adolescent Development ,153 ,23-46, 2016 .   77   4

E. Hoekzema, E. Barba-Müller, C. Pozzobon, M. Picado, F. Lucco, D. García-García, J.-C. Soliva, A. Tobeña, M. Desco, E. Crone, A. Ballesteros, S. Carmona ı O. Vilarroya, "Pregnancy leads to long-lasting changes in human brain structure," Nature Neuroscience ,20 ,287-296, 2017 .   77   5

N. Scott, M. Prigge, O. Yizhar ı T. Kimchi, "A sexually dimorphic hypothalamic circuit controls maternal care and oxytocin secretion," Nature ,525 ,519–522, 2015 .   78   1

Skrundz, M., Bolten, M., Nast, I. et al. Plasma Oxytocin Concentration during Pregnancy is associated with Development of Postpartum Depression. Neuropsychopharmacol 36, 1886–1893 (2011).   80   3

N. Scott, M. Prigge, O. Yizhar ı T. Kimchi, "A sexually dimorphic hypothalamic circuit controls maternal care and oxytocin secretion," Nature ,525 ,519–522, 2015.　81　3

I. Gordon, O. Zagoory-Sharon, J. Leckman ı R. Feldman, "Oxytocin, cortisol, and triadic family interactions," Physiology & Behavior ,5 ,101 ,679-84, 2010 .　82　1

E. Abraham, G. Gilam, Y. Kanat-Maymon, Y. Jacob, O. Zagoory-Sharon, H. Talma ı R. Feldman, "The Human Coparental Bond Implicates Distinct Corticostriatal Pathways: Longitudinal Impact on Family Formation and Child Well-Being," Neuropsychopharmacology ,42 ,2301–2313, 2017 .　82　last

J. E. Swain, P. Kim ı S. S. Ho, "Neuroendocrinology of Parental Response to Baby-Cry," Journal of Neuroendocrinology ,11 ,23 ,1036–1041, 2011 .　83　2

K. Pilyoung, P. Rigo, L. Mayes, R. Feldman, J. Leckman ı J. Swain, "Neural plasticity in fathers of human infants," Social Neuroscience Vol. 9 2014　83　3

Patricia Schreiner-Engel, Raul C. Schiavi, Daniel White, Anna Ghizzani, Low sexual desire in women: The role of reproductive hormones, Hormones and Behavior, Volume 23, Issue 2, 1989, Pages 221-234　84　4

Meston C. M. & Buss D. M. (2009). Why women have sex: understanding sexual motivations from adventure to revenge (and everything in between) (1st ed.). Times Books.　86　last

S. W. Porges, The Polyvagal Theory: Neurophysiological Foundations of Emotions, Attachment, Communication, and Self-Regulation, Barnes and Noble, 2011 .　87　3

E. Lisitsa, "The Four Horsemen: Criticism, Contempt, Defensiveness, and Stonewalling," The Gottman Institute, 2013.　88　4

https://www.mako.co.il/news-lifestyle/2020_q1/Article-164bae7a2db7071027.htm　92　4

World Population Review, "Divorce Rate By State 2021," World Population Review.　92　5

F. A. Beach ı L. Jordan, "Sexual exhaustion and recovery in the male rat," The Quarterly Journal of Experimental Psychology ,8 ,121–133, 1956 .　93　4

G. L. Lester ı B. B. Gorzalka, "Effect of novel and familiar mating partners on the duration of sexual receptivity in the female hamster," Behavioral and Neural Biology ,3 ,49 ,398-405, 1988 .　95　2

B. Phillips-Farfán, M. Romano-Torres ı A. Fernández-Guasti, "Anabolic androgens restore mating after sexual satiety in male rats," Pharmacology, Biochemistry and Behavior ,89 ,241–246, 2007 .　97　1

E. Koukounas ı R. Over, "Habituation of male sexual arousal: effects of attentional focus," Biological Psychology ,1 ,58 ,49-64, 2001 .　98　1

T. Love, C. Laier, M. Brand, L. Hatch ı R. Hajela, "Neuroscience of Internet Pornography Addiction: A Review and Update," Behavioral Sciences ,3 ,5 ,, 388–433, 2015 .　98　last

R. F. Baumeister, "Gender differences in erotic plasticity: The female sex drive as socially flexible and responsive," Psychological Bulletin ,3 ,126 ,347–374, 2000 .　99　1

M. Ketchiff, "Infidelity Survey: What Cheating Looks Like," Shape.com, 201　100　1

S. C. Griffith ı S. Immler, "Female Infidelity and Genetic Compatibility in Birds: The Role of the Genetically Loaded Raffle in Understanding the Function of Extrapair Paternity," Journal of Avian Biology ,2 ,40 ,97-101, 2009 .　100　2

R. Dawkins, The Selfish Gene, Oxford University Press, USA, 1976 .　102　2

S. Pappas, "Genetic testing and family secrets," American Psychological Association ,6 ,49 , 44, 2018 .　102　3

W. Arndt, J. Foehl ı E. Good, "Specific Sexual Fantasy Themes: A Multidimensional Study," Journal of Personality and Social Psychology, ,48,2 , 472-480, 1985 .　104　last

R. F. Baumeister, Social Psychology and Human Sexuality, Routledge, 2001.　104　last

Sapolsky, R. M. (2001). A primate's memoir. A Neuroscientist's Unconventional Life Among the Baboons, New York, Scribner.　105　2

Heske, E. J.; Nelson, RJ (1984). "Pregnancy interruption in Microtus ochrogaster: Laboratory artifact or field phenomenon?". Biology of Reproduction. 31 (1): 97–103.　105　last

B. G. Dias ı K. J. Ressler, "Parental olfactory experience influences behavior and neural structure in subsequent generations," Nature Neuroscience ,17 ,89–96, 2014 .　106　3

Jablonka, Eva; Lamb, Marion J.; Avital, Eytan (1998). "'Lamarckian' mechanisms in Darwinian evolution". Trends in Ecology & Evolution. 13 (5): 206–210.　107　2

https://en.wikipedia.org/wiki/Parthenogenesis　108　1

N. P. Hemanth ı L. J. Young, "Vasopressin and pair-bond formation: genes to brain to behavior," Physiology, 146-52, 2006 .　111　last

E. Amadei, Z. Johnson, Y. J. Kwon, A. Shpiner, V. Saravanan, W. Mays, S. Ryan, H. Walum, D. Rainnie, L. Young ı R. Liu, "Dynamic corticostriatal activity biases social bonding in monogamous female prairie voles," Nature ,7957 ,546 ,, 297–301, 2017 .　113　last

A. Bendesky, Y.-M. Kwon, J.-M. Lassance, C. L. Lewarch, S. Yao, B. K. Peterson, M. X. He, C. Dulac ı H. E. Hoekstra, "The genetic basis of parental care evolution in monogamous mice," Nature ,544 ,434–439, 2017 .　114　2

H. Fujii-Hanamoto, K. Matsubayashi, M. Nakano, H. Kusunoki ı T. Enomoto, "A comparative study on testicular microstructure and relative sperm production in gorillas, chimpanzees, and orangutans," American Hournal of Primatology ,6 ,73 ,570-577, 2011 .　117　2

R. Baker, Sperm Wars: Infidelity, Sexual Conflict, and Other Bedroom Battles, Basic Books, 2006 .	117	3
M. Jensen-Seaman I L. Wen-Hsiung, "Evolution of the Hominoid Semenogelin Genes, the Major Proteins of Ejaculated Semen," Journal of Molecular Evolution volume 57, 261–270, 2003 .	117	4
Zajenkowski M, Gignac GE, Rogoza R, Górniak J, Maciantowicz O, Leniarska M, Jonason PK, Jankowski KS. Ego-Boosting Hormone: Self-Reported and Blood-Based Testosterone Are Associated with Higher Narcissism. Psychol Sci. 2023 Sep;34(9):1024-1032.	118	2
ZERJAL, T. (2003). The Genetic Legacy of the Mongols. The American Journal of Human Genetics, 72 (3), 717-721	118	3
G. P. Murdock, "Atlas of World Cultures," The University of Pittsburgh Press, 1981 .	119	4
"Monogamy". Encyclopaedia Judaica. Vol. 12. pp. 258–260.	120	
Walum H, Young LJ. The neural mechanisms and circuitry of the pair bond. Nat Rev Neurosci. 2018 Nov;19(11):643-654.	122	1
Rosin, Hanna. 2012. The End of Men and the Rise of Women. New York: Riverhead Books.	125	1
C. Jenkins, What Love Is: And What It Could Be, Basic Books, 2017 .	127	2
Counting for Nothing: What Men Value and What Women are Worth, Marilyn Waring, Dec 1999, University of Toronto Press	130	1
British Social Attitudes Survey, 2022, [on-line] bbc.com/news/uk-66866879	130	2
The Price of Motherhood: Why the Most Important Job in the World Is Still the Least Valued, Ann Crittenden 2010, Picador	130	last
Gottman, J.M., and Carrere, S., (1994). Why can't men and women get along? Developmental roots and marital inequities. In D.J. Canary and L. Stafford (Eds.), Communication and Relational Maintenance, Academic Press, Ch. 10, 203-229;	131	last
N. Shpancer, "How Your Personality Predicts Your Romantic Life," 2016 [on-line] psychologytoday.com.	135	3
I. Schneiderman, O. Zagoory-Sharon, J. F. Leckman I R. Feldman, "Oxytocin during the initial stages of romantic attachment: Relations to couples' interactive reciprocity," Psychoneuroendocrinology 37, 8, 1277–1285, 2012 .	136	2
Wise, R. Dopamine, learning and motivation. Nat Rev Neurosci 5, 483–494	138	1
Chapman, G. D. (2010). The five love languages. Walker Large Print.	139	last
McKinney, K. (2011). The Effects of Adrenaline on Arousal and Attraction. Scholars: McKendree University Online Journal of Undergraduate Research, 17.	141	1
J. A. Roberts I M. E. David, "My life has become a major distraction from my cell phone: Partner phubbing and relationship satisfaction among romantic partners," Computers in Human Behavior, 54, 134-141, 2016 .	142	2
B. T. McDaniel I S. M. Coyne, "Technoference": The interference of technology in couple relationships and implications for women's personal and relational well-being," Psychology of Popular Media Culture 1, 5, 85-98, 2016 .	142	2
Turkle, Sherry. Alone Together: Why We Expect More from Technology and Less From Each Other. New York, Basic Books, 2012	142	last
G. L. Greif I K. H. Deal, Two Plus Two, Couples and their Couple friends, Routledge, 2012 .	143	2
Couples' experiences of sacred sex/Tantra practices, Kruse, Cheryl Lynn. California Institute of Integral Studies ProQuest Dissertations Publishing, 2002.	146	last
The UK Wedding Report 2022	147	last
A healthy sex life – at any age! Harvard Healthbeat Newsletter, 6/4/2010	148	2
sapolsky, R. M. (2017). Behave: The biology of humans at our best and worst. Penguin Books.	149	2
Gottman, J.M., and Rushe, R.H., (1994). Communication and social skills approaches to treating ailing marriages: A recommendation for a new marital therapy called "minimal marital therapy." In W. O'Donahue and L. Krasner (Eds.), Handbook of Psychological Skills Training: Clinical Techniques and Applications, Ch. 13, 287-305;	149	
Gottman, J.M., and Carrere, S., (1994). Why can't men and women get along? Developmental roots and marital inequities. In D.J. Canary and L. Stafford (Eds.), Communication and Relational Maintenance, Academic Press, Ch. 10, 203-229;	149	
The Speech code, Liora Weinbach, Beit Alim Publisher, Hebrew	150	2
Gottman, J. (2000). The seven principles for making marriage work. Orion.	152-4	
K. Hall, "Understanding Validation: A Way to Communicate Acceptance," 2012, [on-line] psychologytoday.com.	154	1
M. B. Rosenberg, "Nonviolent Communication: A Language of Life: Life-Changing Tools for Healthy Relationships," PuddleDancer Press, 2015.	156	3
E. Ricciardi, G. Rota, L. Sani, C. Gentili, A. Gaglianese, M. Guazzelli I P. Pietrini, "How the brain heals emotional wounds: the functional neuroanatomy of forgiveness," Frontiers in Human Neuroscience 7, 839, 2013 .	158	2
C. V. Witvliet, T. E. Ludwig I D. J. Bauer, "Please Forgive Me: Transgressors' Emotions and Physiology During Imagery of Seeking Forgiveness and Victim Responses," Journal of Psychology and Christianity, 21, 219-233, 2002 .	158	3

Hall, Jeffrey. (2017). Humor in romantic relationships: A meta-analysis: Humor meta-analysis. Personal Relationships. 24. 10.1111/pere.12183.	160	2
Gray, John, 1951-. Men Are from Mars, Women Are from Venus: a Practical Guide for Improving Communication and Getting What You Want in Your Relationships. New York, NY: HarperCollins, 1992.	162	1
Gershoni, M., Pietrokovski, S. The landscape of sex-differential transcriptome and its consequent selection in human adults. BMC Biol 15, 7 (2017).	162	3
Brizendine, L. (2006). The female brain. New York, Morgan Road Books.	163	3
Palombit RA. Infanticide as sexual conflict: coevolution of male strategies and female counterstrategies. Cold Spring Harb Perspect Biol. 2015 May 18;7(6):	164	1
R. M. Sapolsky, Why Zebras Don't Get Ulcers: The Acclaimed Guide to Stress, Stress-Related Diseases, and Coping, Holt Paperbacks, 2004 .	165	last
S. Gelstein, Y. Yeshurun, L. Rozenkrantz, S. Shushan, I. Frumin, Y. Roth ו N. Sobel, "Human Tears Contain a Chemosignal," Science ,6014 ,331 ,226-30, 2011 .	166	1
E. Hoekzema, E. Barba-Müller, C. Pozzobon, M. Picado, F. Lucco, D. García-García, J. C. Soliva, A. Tobeña, M. Desco, E. A. Crone, A. Ballesteros, S. Carmona ו O. Vilarroya, "Pregnancy leads to long-lasting changes in human brain structure," Nature Neuroscience ,20 ,287-296, 2017 .	166	last

ACKNOWLEDGEMENTS

"To Maya and Milan – the love of my life,
To my brother and father (RIP) who taught me love
and to the man I love who is always there – Erez"